Pesticides and Human Health

William H. Hallenbeck
Kathleen M. Cunningham-Burns

Pesticides
and
Human Health

Springer-Verlag
New York Berlin Heidelberg Tokyo

WILLIAM H. HALLENBECK
School of Public Health
University of Illinois at Chicago
Chicago, Illinois 60680
U.S.A.

KATHLEEN M. CUNNINGHAM-BURNS
School of Public Health
University of Illinois at Chicago
Chicago, Illinois 60680
U.S.A.

Library of Congress Cataloging in Publication Data
Hallenbeck, William H.
   Pesticides and Human Health
   Includes bibliographies and index.
   1. Pesticides—Toxicology.   I. Cunningham-Burns,
Kathleen M.   II. Title.   [DNLM: 1. Pesticides—adverse
effects.   2. Pesticides—toxicology. WA 240 H18p]
RA1270.P4H34   1985   615.7   84-20275

Typeset by University Graphics, Inc., Atlantic Highlands, New Jersey.
Printed and bound by R. R. Donnelley & Sons, Harrisonburg, Virginia.
Printed in the United States of America.

9 8 7 6 5 4 3 2 1

ISBN 0-387-96050-3 Springer-Verlag New York Berlin Heidelberg Tokyo
ISBN 3-540-96050-3 Springer-Verlag Berlin Heidelberg New York Tokyo

To Walter and Carolyn

Preface

The impetus for this book came from numerous requests by public and private agencies and citizens for information regarding the human health effects of pesticide exposures. We have tried to compile a relatively complete, concise summary of the acute and chronic health effects and the toxicology of pesticides in a format that provides quick and easy access. This book was written to address the needs of the following groups: medical and public health professionals, toxicologists, environmentalists, industrial hygienists, regulators, producers and users of pesticides, public interest advocates, and the legal profession.

Acknowledgments

We are indebted to Mr. Christopher J. Wiant, Chief of the Environmental Chemistry Section of the Illinois Department of Public Health. The financial support provided by his office was essential in producing this book.

We are also indebted to Dr. Charles Benbrook, former staff member, and Representative George E. Brown, Chairman of the Subcommittee on Department Operations, Research and Foreign Agriculture of the Committee on Agriculture, United States House of Representatives, for their guidance in obtaining pesticide toxicity data. In the Freedom of Information Office, Office of Pesticide Programs of the United States Environmental Protection Agency, the patience and assistance of Therese Murtagh and Virginia Salzman in obtaining documents are appreciated.

Of the numerous individuals who participated in the production of this book, the following merit special recognition for the quality of their research, editing, and critical skills: Mark Loafman, Sue Ramirez, Steve Smith, Sally Burns, and Denise Steurer.

Finally, we acknowledge the contributions made by those researchers and health workers who have devoted their time and energy to the identification and understanding of the health effects that are summarized in this book.

Contents

Introduction

This book provides a relatively complete summary of the human health effects of pesticide exposures. It contains a compilation of information from numerous sources including texts, government documents, and journals.

The health effects information is organized into the following categories: Acute Exposure Effects, Chronic Exposure Effects, Suspected Effects, and Toxicology. These categories are discussed at the end of the introduction (see Format of Health Information).

Some pesticide ingredients[a] have been placed in classes based on similar chemical structure, toxic mechanisms, and human health effects. Not all ingredients could be classified. Therefore an indication is made as to whether the health information refers to a class of ingredients or an individual ingredient.

Inert ingredients, which are not usually treated in discussions of pesticide health effects, have been included in this book. They frequently comprise a large percentage of a commercial pesticide product, and their adverse effects may exceed those of the active ingredients. For example, carbon tetrachloride and chloroform, both potent liver and central nervous system toxins, are used as inert ingredients without warning on the product label (there is no requirement that inert ingredients be specified on pesticide labels). In cases of poisoning, information regarding the composition of the inert ingredients used in a product should be obtained from the manufacturer to accurately assess the potential health impact of the exposure. It may be necessary to contact the local poison control center or department of health for assistance in obtaining this information. Health effects of many of the toxic inert ingredients are included in this book. A listing of all inert ingredients appears in the Code of Federal Regulations Title 40, 180.1001.

The sources used in compiling health effects information are listed under References Consulted and Suggested. Those effects that were observed in equivocal human pesticide exposures or animal studies are listed in the category Suspected Effects for each ingredient or class of ingredients and are referenced under References Cited. The reader may find the titles listed under References Consulted and Suggested useful in obtaining additional informa-

[a]Pesticide terminology used in this book is defined in Appendix 1 (Glossary of Selected Terms).

tion on the health effects, toxic mechanisms, chemical composition, formulation, manufacturers, and trade names.

The authors have attempted to use standard terminology throughout this book. However, the reader may wish to refer to Appendix 1 for clarification of pesticide terminology and the following medical terms: mucous membrane effects, prenatal effects, postnatal effects, and reproductive effects.

To present health information regarding pesticides in a concise and readily accessible form, the following simplifications were made:

1. The authors included positive outcomes (the presence of an effect) and excluded negative outcomes (the absence of effects).

2. The discussions of toxicology are abbreviated and limited to information that the authors felt would be useful in understanding pesticide health effects. The complete mechanisms of human toxicity are known for very few pesticide ingredients.

3. Routes of exposure have not been specified because they were often inadequately discussed in the source literature. Also, inert ingredients in pesticides often alter the uptake and effects resulting from an exposure route, e.g., the inert ingredient DMSO may facilitate dermal and membrane penetration of an active ingredient, resulting in effects that are not usually associated with dermal exposure to that active ingredient.

In cases where a distinction was not made between the chronic or acute nature of exposures, the health effects for the ingredients are listed under the general heading Exposure Effects. Information was sometimes unavailable for chronic, genotoxic, subacute, and delayed effects and for newer pesticides. These information gaps occur infrequently and are noted in the text.

Due to the widespread use of pesticides, low-level exposures to numerous pesticide ingredients are common. Pesticides are present in most commercially grown food, are used extensively for residential and commercial building pest control, and may be found in most water supplies. There are gaps in the federal government's efforts to limit exposure to pesticides via food, water, and pest control:

There are drinking water standards for only a few pesticides.

Pesticide use instructions for pest control applicators, farmers, and others may result in undesirable exposure levels because actual use patterns are not routinely monitored.

Food tolerances for pesticides are based on arbitrary safety factors which don't confer the same margin of safety for all pesticides.

Synergisms within and among classes of pesticides are not accounted for in setting exposure standards.

The exposure standard for each active ingredient is determined for that ingredient alone. Consideration is not given to the additive effects of other similar-acting members of the same pesticide class. As a result of this method of safety evaluation, an individual's exposure to a class of pesticides may reach a much higher level than the federally determined safe level for specific members of a class. The exposed individual may suffer adverse health effects following exposure to numerous members of a class of pesticides through diet, water, and ambient air, even though the exposure level for each pesticide was below the federally defined safe tolerance level.

In some cases, the health effects attributed to active ingredients have been obtained from human or animal studies in which exposure to a trade product occurred. Trade products contain active and inert ingredients; however, the inert ingredient composition is proprietary information. Consequently, health effects have been attributed to active ingredients in the literature. In addition, some data sources do not indicate whether exposure to a pure active ingredient or to a trade product produced the effects. It is also common practice to use a technical grade of an active ingredient in health effects studies. Technical grades may contain small amounts of impurities that can induce responses different than those of the pure active ingredient. An historical example of this was the contamination of 2, 4, 5-T with TCDD (dioxin). (This is discussed under Chlorophenoxys.) The authors believe the presence of inert ingredients and/or impurities in active ingredients have confounded the effects of relatively few pesticide ingredients discussed in this book.

FORMAT OF
HEALTH INFORMATION

Name

Active or Inert Ingredient or Class

Use: active ingredient uses, e.g., herbicide, insecticide, nematicide

Synonyms: Commonly used names of pesticide ingredients which are not members of a class are listed here. The synonyms of members of a class are listed under the last category, Active and Inert Ingredients.

Composition: The usual chemical compositions are given for those solvents that have varying compositions. The health effects listed are relevant to the composition specified.

Acute Exposure Effects

Health effects that usually result from one or a few exposures to the ingredient(s) are listed in alphabetical order. These effects and those listed under the next two categories (Chronic and Additional Exposure Effects) have been observed in humans following exposure. They do not include experimental data from animal or anecdotal human exposure observations. Some health effects are grouped by the system affected, e.g., respiratory: dyspnea, pulmonary edema. Both signs and symptoms are included in all four effects categories (Acute, Chronic, Additional, and Suspected Effects). When the cause of death is clearly established, it is listed last. Unless otherwise noted, effects occur shortly after exposure.

Chronic Exposure Effects

Health effects that usually result from repeated low-level exposures as in an occupational or environmental setting are listed in this category. Due to individual variations in susceptibilities and response, effects usually associated with acute exposure may be observed following chronic exposures and vice versa.

Additional Exposure Effects of Members of a Class
Individual members of a class may cause effects that have not been associated with the entire class. These are listed by ingredient in alphabetical order.

Suspected Effects
Effects listed in this category are derived from animal studies or equivocal human exposures. These effects usually include carcinogenesis, mutagenesis, pre- and postnatal damage, reproductive system damage, and other outcomes that are difficult to link unequivocally with a particular agent. This category is especially important for newer pesticides, which have been the subject of government-mandated animal studies but often have little human exposure information. Suspected effects are followed by reference numbers and, where applicable, page numbers in parentheses. Suspected effects of a class are listed first, followed by suspected effects of individual members of the class.

Toxicology
A succinct summary of physiological interactions are given in this section. Additional data on the toxicology of individual members of a class are listed below the class toxicology.

Additional Information
This category contains miscellaneous health-related information that may be useful to the reader.

Active and Inert Ingredients
The names of the active and inert ingredients in a class and their synonyms appear in this category. When synonyms are listed, they are followed by the most commonly used ingredient name in parentheses. For example, EDB is followed by (ethylene dibromide). Some trade names have been included because they are commonly used to refer to specific active ingredients.

Note
THE READER IS URGED TO USE CAUTION in evaluating the relationship between pesticides and health effects. Individual variations in response exist. Consequently, exposure victims may manifest only some or none of the effects listed. In addition, effects not listed may be exhibited.

Acetanilides

Class of Active Ingredients

Use: fungicides, herbicides

Acute Exposure Effects

abdominal distress
acetanilide in urine
p-aminophenol
  metabolite in urine
anemia
ataxia
blood: brown
chills
collapse
convulsions

cyanosis
dermal: irritation,
  dermatitis,
  sensitization
diarrhea
eye irritation
GI irritation
indophenol test
  positive
jaundice

mucous membrane
  irritation
muscular weakness
nausea
shock
sweating
urine: dark
vomiting

Death due to CNS
  depression

Chronic Exposure Effects

anemia
collapse
dermal: dermatitis,
  sensitization
dizziness

dyspnea
hepatic damage
mucous membrane
  irritation

nephritis

Death due to circulatory
  or respiratory failure

Suspected Effects

Alachlor:
carcinogenesis 23
ocular lesions 23
postnatal damage 23
prenatal damage 23
Butachlor:
mutagenesis 23
Carboxin:
corneal opacities 29(44)
dermal edema 29(45)
renal degeneration 29(41)

Metolachlor:
corneal opacities 23
prenatal damage 23
Propachlor:
mutagenesis 27
Propanil:
methemoglobinemia 9(538)
mutagenesis due to the metabolite
  3,4-dichloroaniline 22, 27

Toxicology

Propanil effects may be potentiated by organophosphates and carbamates. Acetanilides degrade to aniline derivatives.

Additional Information
Cardiac patients are especially susceptible to the toxic effects of acetanilides.

Active Ingredients

alachlor

butachlor

carboxin

metolachlor

oxycarboxin

propachlor

propanil

Acetone _____

Inert Ingredient

Synonym: dimethyl ketone

Acute Exposure Effects

acetone levels in blood greater than 2 mg/dl
bronchitis
carbohydrate metabolism altered
CNS dysfunction and depression
collapse
convulsions
coughing
dermatitis
dizziness
drowsiness
eye: irritation, conjunctivitis, corneal erosion
fainting attacks
gastrititis
headache
hematemesis
mucous membrane irritation
muscle weakness
nausea
restlessness
rhinorrhea
stupor
twitching
unconsciousness
urine: positive Ketostix reading

Chronic Exposure Effects
Chronic effects may exist, but no data were found.

Suspected Effects
mutagenesis 27

Toxicology
Acetone is a fat solvent that causes CNS dysfunction and destruction of other tissues. It stimulates cytochrome P-450-mediated oxidations. It can potentiate carbon tetrachloride hepatotoxicity.

Acetonitrile ───────────────────────────

Inert Ingredient

Synonyms: cyanomethane, ethanenitrile, methyl cyanide

Acute Exposure Effects
See Cyanides for additional effects.

abdominal pain
chest tightness and
  pain
coma
convulsions
cyanide in blood
delirium
dermal irritation

eye irritation
flushing of face
GI disturbance
hematemesis
metabolic acidosis
mucous membrane
  irritation

nausea
paralysis
respiratory depression
shock
thiocyanates in urine
unconsciousness

Chronic Exposure Effects
See Cyanides for additional effects.

dermatitis
dizziness
headache
weakness

Suspected Effects
ataxia 27
corneal damage 27
dyspnea 27

Toxicology
Acetonitrile is metabolized to hydrogen cyanide, which is slowly released and concentrates in the brain, heart, kidney, and spleen (see Cyanides). It complexes with metal in enzymes, causing cessation of cellular respiration. It can penetrate skin.

Individuals with a history of fainting spells or convulsions are especially susceptible.

Following inhalation or ingestion, there is usually a latent period of several hours before symptoms appear.

Acrolein ——————————————————————

Active Ingredient

Use: algicide, fumigant, herbicide, slimicide

Acute Exposure Effects

abdominal pain
allergic hypersensitivity
burning sensation in nose and
  throat
CNS depression
convulsions
cyanosis
dermal: burns, dermatitis,
  sensitization
diarrhea
dizziness
drowsiness
eye: irritation, tearing,
  conjunctivitis, double vision
GI upset
headache

mucous membrane irritation
muscle weakness
nausea
respiratory: bronchitis,
  bronchospasm, dyspnea,
  hoarseness, substernal pressure,
  coughing of frothy sputum,
  pulmonary and laryngeal edema,
  respiratory depression
tremor
unconsciousness
vomiting
wheezing

Death due to pulmonary edema or
  respiratory failure

Chronic Exposure Effects
dermal: dermatitis, burns, sensitization (rash, hives)

Suspected Effects
carcinogenesis 26
fatty liver 26
metaplasia and hyperplasia in
  trachea and nasal cavity 20

mutagenesis 27
prenatal damage 27

Alcohols (Aliphatic) ──────────────────

Class of Inert Ingredients

Exposure Effects

acidosis
alcohol in expired air, urine, and
   blood
ataxia
cardiac arrhythmias
CNS depression
coma
confusion
convulsions
delirium
dermal irritation
diarrhea
dizziness
eye irritation
fatigue
giddiness

GI hemorrhage
glycosuria
headache
hepatic damage
nausea
renal damage
respiratory disorders: cough,
   irritation, dyspnea, pulmonary
   edema, respiratory depression
unconsciousness
vomiting
weakness
weight loss

Death due to respiratory
   or cardiac failure

Additional Exposure Effects of Individual Aliphatic Alcohols

n-Butanol:
   conjunctivitis
   keratitis
   mucous membrane irritation
   vertigo
Ethanol:
   Babinski sign
   gastroenteritis
   Korsakoff's syndrome
   mental deterioration
   sensory loss
   tremors
   visual disturbances
Ethylene Glycol:
   albuminuria
   anuria
   cyanosis
   hematuria
   lymphocytosis
   meningoencephalitis
   oxalic acid in urine
   tremors

Isopropanol:
   anemia
   anuria
   hypotension
   uremia
Methanol:
   abdominal pain
   albuminuria
   blindness
   conjunctivitis
   cyanosis
   formaldeyde and formic acid in
      urine
   hypotension
   mydriasis
   numbness in limbs
   sweating

Toxicology

Alcohols are metabolized by a common enzyme system, alcohol dehydrogenase, to their corresponding aldehydes, ketones, and acids. Primary alcohols are oxidized to their corresponding aldehydes and acids. Secondary alcohols are metabolized to ketones, which are CNS depressants. Tertiary alcohols are metabolized slowly and incompletely, and their effects are especially persistent.

Aliphatic alcohols potentiate the toxicity of halogenated hydrocarbons such as chloroform and carbon tetrachloride.

Inert Ingredients

n-butanol

ethanol

ethylene glycol

ispropanol

methanol

Amitrole

Active Ingredient

Synonym: aminotriazole
Use: herbicide

Suspected Effects

antithyroid effects resulting in
  goiter 3(2703), 9(565–6), 36
carcinogenesis 1, 3(2703), 9(565–6),
  20, 26, 27, 28, 36
hemorrhage 9(564)
hyperperistalsis 9(564)

mutagenesis 27
postnatal damage 9(566), 27
prenatal damage 3(2704), 27
pulmonary edema 9(564)
spleen atrophy 9(566)

Other effects may occur, but no data were found.

Toxicology

Amitrole inhibits: catalases in the liver and kidneys, peroxidase, thyroid uptake of iodine, δ-aminolevulinic acid dehydratase, and cytochrome P-450.

Ammonium Sulfamate ──────────────

Active Ingredient

Use: herbicide

Acute Exposure Effects

bradypnea	dermal irritation	nausea
coma	eye irritation	prostration
convulsions	GI irritation	vomiting

Other effects may occur, but no data were found.

Anticoagulants —————————————————————

Class of Active Ingredients

Use: rodenticides

Acute Exposure Effects
anemia
abdominal pain
back pain
capillary wall destruction
dermal: necrosis; petechial rash;
  ecchymoses; hematomas of skin,
  joints, and buttocks
hematologic disorders
hematuria
melena

hemorrhage: mucous membrane,
  lips, gums, nose
pallor
paralysis due to cerebral
  hemorrhage
prothrombin depression
renal colic
weakness

Death due to hermorrhagic shock

Chronic Exposure Effects
Same as above

Suspected Effects
prenatal damage 4(A-92), 5(171), 23

Toxicology
Anticoagulants are antimetabolites of vitamin K and inhibit the synthesis of prothrombin.

Additional Information
Symptoms may not appear for a few days or weeks. Repeated exposure is usually required for damage to occur. Numerous small exposures may be more damaging than one large exposure.

Active Ingredients
brodifacoum
bromadiolone
chlorophacinone
coumachlor
coumafene (warfarin)

coumafuryl
coumatetralyl
Dicumarol®
difenacoum
diphacinone

pindone
2-pivalyl-1,3-
  indandione
  (pindone)
warfarin

ANTU

Active Ingredient

> **Synonym:** 1-naphthylthiourea
> **Use:** rodenticide

Acute Exposure Effects

cyanosis
dyspnea
eczema

pulmonary rales
vomiting

Chronic Exposure Effects

Chronic effects may exist, but no data were found.

Suspected Effects

antiadrenal activity 1
antithyroid activity 8(III–38)
anuria/oliguria 8(III–38)
carcinogenesis 1, 26, 27
hepatic glycogen depletion 8(III–38)
hydrothorax 8(III–38)

hyperglycemia 8(III–38)
hypothermia 8(III–39)
mutagenesis 9(506), 11(354), 27
pleural effusion 8(III–38), 9(506)
pulmonary edema 8(III–38), 9(506)

Additional Information

ANTU may contain the impurity β-naphthylamine, which is a carcinogen.

Arsenicals

Class of Active Ingredients

Use: fungicides, herbicides, insecticides, rodenticides

Acute Exposure Effects

abdominal pain, burning, dehydration

arsenic in stomach contents, urine, hair, skin, bone, and liver

capillary permeability increase

bowel dehydration and pain

chills

clammy skin

CNS injury

colic

collapse

coma

convulsions

cramps

cyanosis

delirium

dermal: dermatitis (exfoliative), edema (eyelid, facial)

diarrhea: bloody, watery, mucous, painful

dizziness

dysphagia

EKG abnormalities

electrolyte loss

encephalopathy

esophageal pain

garlic odor: breath and feces

gastroenteritis (hemorrhagic)

giddiness

goiter

headache

hematemesis

hemoglobinemia

hemolysis

hepatic: hepatomegaly, jaundice, hepatitis, elevated SGOT and LDH

hyperthermia

mania

melena

metallic taste

mucous membrane irritation

muscle spasms

nausea

paralysis

peripheral neuropathy

pulse feeble

prostration

renal/urinary: nephrosis, tubular necrosis, azotemia, cylindruria, pyuria, albuminuria, anuria/ oliguria, hematuria, hemoglobinuria

respiratory: bronchitis, cough with foamy sputum, pulmonary edema, dyspnea, pneumonia, chest pain, rales, respiratory depression

restlessness

shock

thirst

tongue soreness

vertigo

weakness

Death due to fluid and electrolyte loss

Chronic Exposure Effects

abdominal distress
anemia (aplastic)
anesthesia
anorexia
apathy
arsenic in stomach contents, urine,
  hair, nails, skin, liver, and bone
ataxia
axonal degeneration
bone marrow depression
cold sensations in extremities
dermal: ulceration, pigmentation,
  eczema, keratosis, exfoliation,
  dermatitis, vesiculation,
  sensitization, edema (eyelid), hair
  loss, and cancer
diarrhea/constipation
disorientation
dysphasia
EKG abnormalities
encephalopathy
eye: keratitis, neuritis, and
  conjunctivitis
fatigue
garlic breath
GI disturbance
headache
hepatic: hepatitis, hepatomegaly,
  jaundice, cirrhosis, elevated
  SGOT and LDH, carcinogenesis
hypesthesia
hypersusceptibility to infection
hyperthermia

motor neuron conduction velocity
  depression
muscular atrophy
nails: brittle, deformed, loss,
  horizontal white bands
nasal obstruction and necrosis of
  cartilage with perforation
nausea
neuralgia
pallor
pancytopenia
paralysis
paresis
paresthesias
peripheral neuropathy
renal/urinary: nephritis, tubular
  necrosis, albuminuria, anuria,
  azotemia, pyuria
respiratory: carcinogenesis,
  bronchitis, pneumonia, cough,
  coryza, laryngitis, pharyngitis,
  rhinitis
salivation
stomatitis
sweating
ulceration of lips, nostrils, eyelids,
  nasal septum, pharynx, scrotum
vertigo
weakness
weight loss

Death due to cardiac fibrillation and
  arrest

Suspected Effects

mutagenesis 7(20), 22
portal hypertension 7(19)
prenatal damage 4(A–44), 5(437),
  7(20), 22

Cacodylic Acid:
mutagenesis 22
reproductive system effects 22

OBPA:
adrenal congestion 35(29)
corneal opacity 35(32)
eye discharge (bloody) 35(30)
pulmonary hemorrhage 35(31)
renal congestion 35(29)
rhinorrhea (bloody) 35(29)
tremors 35(30)
urinary incontinence 35(30)

Toxicology

Trivalent forms are more toxic than pentavalent forms, including pentavalent organics.

Arsenicals:
—are metabolized to arsenite;
—inhibit sulfhydryl enzymes;
—uncouple oxidative and substrate level phosphorylation;
—inhibit pyruvate and α-ketoglutarate dehydrogenase systems;
—inhibit the function of 6,8-dithiooctanoic acid;
—combine with the sulfur of keratin;
—coagulate protein.

Additional Information

Symptoms of arsenical poisoning can be delayed for minutes or hours after exposure.

Active Ingredients

ammonium arsonate
arsenic acid
arsenic pentoxide
arsenic trioxide
cacodylic acid
calcium acid methane arsonate
calcium arsenate
calcium arsenite
calcium arsonate
CAMA (calcium acid methane arsonate)
copper acetoarsenate
copper aceto-meta-arsenite (Paris green)
copper arsenite
dimethylarsinic acid (cacodylic acid)
disodium methanearsonate
dodecylammonium methanearsonate
DSMA (disodium methanearsonate)
lead arsenate
MAA (methane arsonic acid)
MAMA (monoammonium methane arsonate)
methane arsonic acid
monoammonium methane arsonate
monosodium methanearsonate
MSMA (monosodium methane arsonate)
OBPA
Paris green
sodium arsenate
sodium arsenite
sodium arsonate
white arsenic (arsenic trioxide)

Benzene

Inert Ingredient

Acute Exposure Effects
anesthesia
anorexia
ataxia
bone marrow depression
CNS excitement followed by
   depression
coma
confusion
convulsions
delirium
dermal: erythema, edema, pallor,
   dermatitis, flushing, vesciculation
dizziness
drowsiness
erythromyelosis
euphoria followed by fatigue
eye irritation
flushing
hallucinations
headache
hemorrhage

mucous membrane irritation
muscle twitching
nausea
phenolics and glucuronides in urine
respiratory: dyspnea, chest
   constriction, respiratory
   depression, pulmonary edema
   and hemorrhage, pneumonitis
restlessness
tachycardia
tinnitus
tremor
unconsciousness
vertigo
vision blurred
vomiting
weakness

Death due to respiratory failure and
   ventricular fibrillation

Chronic Exposure Effects
anorexia
blood dyscrasias: aplastic anemia,
   erythroleukemia,
   hyperbilirubinemia,
   pancytopenia, leukemia (myeloid
   and lymphatic); leukocytosis,
   thrombocytosis, and
   erythrocytosis followed by
   leukocytopenia,
   thrombocytopenia, and anemia
cardiac sensitization
chromosome aberrations
CNS injury
dizziness
drowsiness
dyspnea
fatigue
headache
hearing impairment

hemolysis
hemorrhage (internal)
hepatic damage
hyperplastic and hypoplastic bone
   marrow
hypotension
iron metabolism disturbed
myocardial changes
nervousness
pallor
polyneuritis
rash
spleno-adrenomegaly
tachycardia
unconsciousness
vertigo
visual disturbances

Death due to respiratory arrest

Suspected Effects

bronchiogenic carcinoma 7(247)

Hodgkin's disease 5(486)

lymphosarcoma 5(486)

malignant lymphoma 7(247)

multiple myeloma 7(247)

mutagenesis 27

myeloid metaplasia 7(247)

myocardial sensitization to
  epinephrine 8(III–321)

paroxysmal nocturnal
  hemoglobinuria 7(247)

prenatal damage 5(168), 27

postnatal damage 27

reproductive system damage 5(343)

Toxicology

Benzene is a fat solvent that causes CNS dysfunction and destruction of other tissues. It is oxidized to phenol, which may inhibit erythrocyte development. Benzene's interaction with DNA may be the cause of pancytopenia and leukemia.

Additional Information

Benzene is very volatile and may exist at much higher concentrations in vapors than in the solvents that were the source of the benzene vapors.

Benzoic Acids ————————————————

Class of Active and Inert Ingredients

Use: herbicides

Acute Exposure Effects

benzoic acid in urine
cyanosis
dyspnea
exhaustion

eye irritation
muscular spasms
urinary incontinence

Chronic Exposure Effects
Chronic exposure effects may exist, but no data were found.

Additional Exposure Effect of DCPA
dermatitis

Suspected Effects
Chloramben:

ataxia 23
carcinogenesis 22, 23, 26, 30(109)
hyperemia (adrenal, pulmonary,
  renal) 30(108)
mutagenesis 23
polyuria 23
prenatal damage 23
ptosis 23
reproductive system effects 22
weight gain depression 22

Dicamba:

ataxia 23
bradycardia 22
bradypnea 23
hyperactivity/sedation 23
prenatal damage 23

Toxicology
Benzoic acids are weak to moderately active inhibitors of the Krebs cycle. However, this is not a primary mode of action.

Additional Information
Benzoic acids are commonly formulated with 2,4-D or MCPA.

Active and Inert Ingredients

benzoic acid	inert ingredient
chloramben	active ingredient
chlorthiamid	active ingredient
DCPA	active ingredient
dicamba	active ingredient
fenac	active ingredient
TBA	active ingredient
TCBA (TBA)	active ingredient
terephthalic acid (DCPA)	active ingredient
2,3,6-trichlorobenzoic acid (TBA)	active ingredient

Benzonitriles ━━━━━━━━━━━━━━━━━━━━━━━━━━━━

Class of Active Ingredients

Use: fungicides, herbicides

Ioxynil
Acute Exposure Effects:
  hyperemia of all organs
  edema of the lungs and brain

Ioxynil and Bromoxynil
Chronic Exposure Effects:

dizziness
elevation (transient) of aldolase,
   creatinine phosphokinase, LDH,
   and SGOT
headache
hyperthermia

muscle pain
sweating
thirst
vomiting
weakness
weight loss

Dichlobenil
Acute and Chronic Exposure Effects:
  dermatitis

Suspected Effects:
  anorexia 23
  hematuria 23
  hepatomegaly 9(541), 23
  jaundice 23
  leukocyte infiltration around central
     veins 23
  postnatal damage 23
  renal hypertrophy 9(541), 23
  reproductive system effects 23

Chlorothalonil
Acute Exposure Effects:
  dermatitis, eye irritation

Suspected Effects:
  ataxia 23
  carcinogenesis 11(326)
  dermal: edema, erythema,
     sensitization 23
  DNA repair interference 23

growth suppression 22, 23
postnatal damage 23, 36
prenatal damage 22, 23
renal: hypertrophy, nephritis 23, 36

Toxicology

Toxicity may be due to the uncoupling of oxidative phosphorylation and inhibition of electron transport.

Chlorothalonil inhibits specific NAD-thiol dependent glycolytic and respiratory enzymes.

Dichlobenil is frequently mixed with dalapon or bromacil.

Active Ingredients

bromoxynil

bromoxynil octanoate

chlorothalonil

dichlobenil

ioxynil

Bipyridyls _____

Class of Active Ingredients

Use: herbicides

Exposure Effects

dehydration
dermal: irritation, erythema,
    discoloration, fingernail softening
    and loss
diarrhea
dysphagia
hematemesis
hemorrhage (brain, nose)
hepatic: necrosis, jaundice, fatty;
    elevated serum GOT, GPT,
    LDH, and alkaline phosphatase
mucous membrane irritation and
    ulceration (oral, pharyngeal,
    esophageal, gastroenteric)

nausea
renal/urinary: tubular necrosis,
    albuminuria, pyuria, anuria/
    oliguria; elevated serum BUN
    and creatinine
respiratory: irritation, chest pain,
    hyaline membrane formation,
    cough, pulmonary edema,
    hemorrhage

Death due to renal failure

Additional Exposure Effects of Individual Bipyridyls

Diquat:

gastoenteric congestion
lung consolidation
weight loss

Paraquat:

abdominal pain
adrenal necrosis
anorexia
convulsions
cyanosis
EKG disturbances
eye: conjunctivitis, corneal opacity
gastroenteritis
hypotension
myocarditis
peripheral nerve degeneration
respiratory: loss of surfactant,
    proliferation of connective tissue
    in alveolar space, dyspnea,
    inflammatory infiltrates,
    pulmonary fibrosis (rapid and
    progressive)
rhinorrhagia
smooth muscle atrophy
spleen hemorrhage
stomatitis

Additional Exposure Effects of Individual Bipyridyls (*continued*)

Paraquat (*continued*)
tachycardia
vomiting

Death due to cardiac, hepatic, or
respiratory failure

Suspected Effects
Diquat:
anorexia 3(2752)
cataracts 1, 9(559), 23
convulsions 3(2753)
dermal thickening, scabbing 9(559)
dyspnea 3(2752)
dystrophic changes in the heart
3(2755)
GI distension 5(391)
hyperexcitability 5(391)
hypothermia 3(2752)
light reflex absent 3(2752)
lung cell swelling and
desquamation 9(559)
muscle twitching 3(2753)
mutagenesis 27
prenatal damage 3(2756), 9(560),
23, 27
reproductive system effects 5(343)
thickening of interalveolar septa
and peribronchial lymph tissue
9(559), and inflammatory
changes in peribronchial and
perivascular connective tissue
3(2755)

Paraquat:
ataxia 9(543)
convulsions 9(543)
hyperexcitability 9(543)
mutagenesis 27
postnatal damage 3(2755,2756)
prenatal damage 3(2756), 5(401), 27
reproductive system effects 5(343)
tearing 3(2752)
weight loss 9(543)

Toxicology
Bipyridyls are metabolized to free radicals that may deplete NADPH and damage cell membranes.

Additional Information
Bipyridyl symptoms may be delayed 3–14 days.

Active Ingredients
diquat
diquat dibromide
(diquat)

paraquat
paraquat dichloride
(paraquat)

Boric Acid _____

Inert and Active Ingredient

Synonym: boracic acid
Use: fungicide, herbicide, insecticide

Acute Exposure Effects
anorexia
blistering
blood: elevated protein, red blood
   cells, and epithelial casts
boric acid in urine, brain, lung,
   liver
CNS: congestion, stimulation
   followed by depression
coagulation (intravascular)
coma
confusion
convulsions
cyanosis
delirium
dermal: erythematous eruption of
   skin progressing to exfoliative
   dermatitis (usually on palms,
   soles, buttocks, and scrotum),
   leukocytic infiltration, focal
   hemorrhage, red rash, flushing
drowsiness
eye irritation
GI: pain, hemorrhage
headache

hepatic: jaundice, hepatomegaly
hyperthermia
hypotension (arterial)
insomnia
lethargy
meningismus
metabolic acidosis
mucous membrane irritation
muscle spasms
nausea
prostration
pulse: thready
renal/urinary: anuria/oliguria,
   albuminuria, tubular necrosis,
   azotemia
restlessness
shock
tachycardia
tremors
vomiting
weakness

Death due to CNS depression,
   circulatory collapse, or renal failure.

Chronic Exposure Effects
abdominal discomfort
allergic reactions
anemia: hypoplastic
anorexia
CNS congestion
convulsions
dermal: dermatitis, skin atrophy,
   red rash, dryness, eruption, focal
   hemorrhage, leukocytic
   infiltration, hair loss, cracked lips
diarrhea (mild)

digestion disturbances
eye: conjunctivitis, eyelid edema
gastric ulcer
hepatic: degeneration, jaundice
joint pains
meningismus
metabolic acidosis
mucous membrane irritation,
   atrophy, eruptions, dryness
nausea
renal: kidney tubule degeneration

Chronic Exposure Effects (*continued*)

tongue: red

vomiting

weakness

weight loss

Suspected Effects

ataxia 9(62)

mutagenesis 27

prenatal damage
   5(168)

reproductive system
   effects 27

Toxicology

Boric acid is rapidly absorbed from the GI tract and skin. It acts on the nervous system, enzyme systems, carbohydrate metabolism, kidneys, liver, hormone functions, and cellular oxidation. Infants are more susceptible to boric acid than adults. The onset of symptoms may be delayed for hours in acute poisoning.

Carbamates ────────────────────────────────

Class of Active Ingredients

Use: fungicides, herbicides, insecticides, molluscicides, nematicides, plant growth regulators

Acute Exposure Effects

abdominal cramps
aphasia
ataxia
bradycardia
cholinesterase depression
coma
convulsions
cyanosis
dermal irritation
diarrhea
disorientation
dizziness
epigastric pain
eye: pain, blurred vision, loss of accommodation, dim vision, miosis/mydriasis, tearing, ciliary muscle spasm, unreactive pupils
headache
hypertension
incontinence
lassitude
muscle twitching

nausea
pallor
paralysis of extremities (temporary)
psychosis
reflexes abnormal
respiratory: pulmonary edema, cough, chest tightness, dyspnea, rales, oronasal discharge, bronchoconstriction
salivation
sleeping difficulty
sweating
tachycardia
tremor
unconsciousness
vomiting
weakness

Death due to respiratory arrest, respiratory muscle paralysis, or bronchoconstriction

Chronic Exposure Effects

anorexia
cholinesterase depression
muscle weakness

renal/urinary: renal damage, albuminuria, glycosuria

Suspected Effects
  prenatal damage 1, 5(171), 22, 23,
    27, 36
  reproductive system effects 5(343),
    23, 27
Aldicarb:
  N-nitroso derivative is mutagenic
    2(194)
Benomyl
  corneal opacities 23
  hepatic damage 23
  mutagenesis 22, 36
✰*Carbaryl:*
  behavioral effects 36
  carcinogenesis 20, 25
  CNS lesions 8(III–81)
  heart defects 23
  humoral immune response
    suppression 37
  mutagenesis 22
  N-nitroso derivative is carcinogenic
    9(444) and mutagenic 2(193),
    9(444)
  paraplegia 8(III–81)
  prostration 8(III–81)
  renal tubular damage 8(III–80)
  vasogenic edema 8(III–81)
  weight depression 23
Carbofuran:
  N-nitroso derivative is
    mutagenic 2(194)
Chlorpropham:
  carcinogenesis 36
Methomyl:
  adrenal hypertrophy 23
  bone marrow damage 33(87)
  breathing irregular 33(82)
  dermal: edema, erythema 33(95)
  eye: conjunctivitis 33(82), corneal
    opacity 33(95), exophthalmos 23,

Methomyl (*continued*)
  33(82), tearing (bloody) 23,
    33(82)
  hematocrit decrease 23
  hemoglobin decrease 23
  hepatic damage 33(87)
  N-nitroso derivative is mutagenic
    2(194)
  prostrate enlargement 23
  splenic damage 33(79)
Mexacarbate:
  carcinogenesis 36
Phenmedipham:
  anemia 23
  hematocrit decrease 23
  hemoglobin decrease 23
  spleen: histologic
    changes 23
Pirimicarb:
  anemia 23
  blood dyscrasias 23
  carcinogenesis 23, 36
  growth retardation 22, 23
  pituitary hypertrophy 23
  spleen weight changes 23
Propham:
  carcinogenesis 36
Propineb:
  carcinogenesis 36
  goitrogenesis 36
  pituitary enlargement
    36
Propoxur:
  N-nitroso derivative is
    mutagenic 2(194)
Thiophanate-methyl:
  metabolite MBC is
    mutagenic 22

Toxicology

Carbamates cause reversible carbamylation of acetylcholinesterase. This leads to accumulation of acetylcholine at cholinergic neuro-effector junctions, which causes muscarinic and nicotinic effects and impaired CNS function. The carbamyl-enzyme complex dissociates readily, which reduces the duration of toxic effects and limits the time during which the poisoning can be detected. Carbamates are metabolized by the liver and are mild inducers of mixed function oxidases. Carbamates alter several other enzyme systems. CNS depressants potentiate carbamate poisoning. Methomyl is potentiated by carbaryl and ronnel.

Additional Information

There is a rapid disappearance of the less severe exposure effects. Cholinesterase activities usually revert to normal within a few hours. Some carbamates yield metabolites that are measurable in urine up to 48 hours after exposure, e.g., 1-naphthol.

Active Ingredients

aldicarb
aminocarb
aprocarb (propoxur)
asulam
barban
bendiocarb
benomyl
4-benzothienyl-*N*-
   methylcarbamate
bufencarb
carbaryl
carbofuran

chlorpropham
dimetan
dioxacarb
isolan
isoprocarb
m-isopropylphenyl-*N*-
   methyl carbamate
Landrin®
methiocarb
methomyl
mexacarbate
oxamyl

PHC (propoxur)
phencyclocarb
phenmedipham
pirimicarb
promecarb
propham
propineb
propoxur
Pyramat®
Pyrolan®
terbucarb
thiophanate methyl

Carbon Disulfide

Active Ingredient

Use: fumigant

Acute Exposure Effects

abdominal pain
areflexia
ataxia
blood protein abnormalities
CNS depression
coma
convulsions
cyanosis
delirium
dermal: irritation, burns,
    sensitization
diarrhea
disorientation
dizziness
drowsiness
EKG abnormalities
eye: irritation, impairment of color
    vision, corneal opacities, double
    vision, retinal degeneration,
    mydriasis
garlic breath
hallucinations
headache
hepatic damage

hypotension
hypothermia
leg weakness
mania
mucous membrane irritation
narcosis
nausea
neurological disorders
palpitations
paralysis
peripheral nerve degeneration
peripheral vascular collapse
prostration
pulse: weak
renal damage
respiratory: bronchitis,
    bronchospasms, laryngeal edema,
    dyspnea, irritation, depression,
    emphysema
tremor
unconsciousness
vertigo
vomiting

Death due to respiratory failure

Chronic Exposure Effects

anemia (hypochromic)
anorexia
anosmia
aphasia
blood: elevation of albumin, β-
    lipoprotein, cholesterol,
    monocytes
cardiac: arrhythmias,
    atherosclerosis, EKG
    abnormalities, angina pectoris

CNS neuropathy
delirium
dermal sensitization
dizziness
dysphagia
EEG abnormalities
encephalopathy
endocrine disorders: adrenal and
    testicular
exhaustion

Chronic Exposure Effects (*continued*)

eye: blindness, optic and retrobulbar neuritis, retinal hypertension, impaired color and night vision, paralysis of accommodation, scotoma, amblyopia, loss of acuity

gastric disturbances

headache

hematuria

hepatic damage

hypertension/hypotension

hypesthesias

impotence

libido decrease

menstrual disorders

neuromuscular: muscle atrophy, hypertrophy, chorea, weakness, athetosis, paralysis, paresthesia, parkinsonism, peripheral neuropathy, nerve conduction impaired, pain along nerve trunks, ataxia, areflexia (lower extremities)

ovarian disorders

personality changes: manic-depressive psychosis, apathy, hallucinations, irritability, transient excitement, suicidal tendencies, memory loss, insomnia, nightmares

respiratory: bronchitis, emphysema

renal damage

sperm abnormalities

spontaneous abortion

ulcers

vertigo

Death due to circulatory or respiratory failure

Suspected Effects

carcinogenesis 16

fibrinolytic activity reduced in serum 8(III–84)

mutagenesis 27

postnatal damage 27

prenatal damage 4(A–11), 27

pyridoxine deficiency 7(264)

reproductive system effects 4(A–11)

retinal microaneurysms 8(III–84)

Toxicology
Carbon Disulfide:

—is partially metabolized to dithiocarbamate, which chelates polyvalent cations, especially copper; it is also metabolized to inorganic and organic sulfates;

—inhibits copper-containing enzymes such as monoamine oxidase (cerebral) and dopamine-β-oxidase (neural);

—interferes with amino acid and lipoprotein metabolism;

—may induce a pyridoxine deficiency contributing to the development of polyneuropathy;

—causes axonal degeneration;

—inhibits mixed-function oxidases;

—may affect women more than men, regarding neurotoxicity.

Chlormequat ⸻

Active Ingredient

Use: plant regulator

Exposure Effects
CNS changes
respiratory depression

Suspected Effects

anticholinesterase
  effects 36
carcinogenesis 26, 27
mutagenesis 27

prenatal damage 26,
  27,36
reproductive system
  effects 36

Other effects may occur, but no data were found.

Chloroalkyl Thios ─────────────────────────

Class of Active Ingredients

Synonym: dicarboximides, phthalimides
Use: fungicides

Acute Exposure Effects

adipsia
anemia
anorexia/weight loss
cholinesterase activity depression
dermal: irritation, rash,
    sensitization
diarrhea
eye: irritation, conjunctivitis
GI irritation
hematuria
hepatic injury
hypertension
hypothermia
irritability
listlessness
mucous membrane irritation
prostration
protein and urobilinogen in urine
    and blood
renal injury
respiratory: bronchitis, sensitization
rhinorrhagia
ulcers
vomiting

Chronic Exposure Effects

dermal irritation
weight loss

Suspected Effects

Captafol:
carcinogenesis 23
dermatitis 1
mutagenesis 22
prenatal damage 22

Captan:
carcinogenesis 2(172), 9(581),
    11(310), 22, 23
mutagenesis 9(580), 11(310), 22
prenatal damage 5(393), 9(582),
    22

Folpet:
carcinogenesis 23
mutagenesis 3(2709)
prenatal damage 5(393)
splenomegaly 3(2708), 23
thyroid enlargement 3(2708), 23

Toxicology

Chloroalkyl thios inhibit mitochondrial function and uncouple oxidative phosphorylation.

Additional Information

Individuals with a serious protein deficiency are especially susceptible to the effects of chloroalkyl thios.

Active Ingredients
captafol
captan
folpet

Chlorophenoxys ——————————————————————

Class of Active Ingredients

Use: herbicides

Acute Exposure Effects

abdominal pain and tenderness
acidosis
anorexia/weight loss
ataxia
chlorophenoxys in urine
CNS damage
coma
convulsions
creatinuria
dermatitis
diarrhea
dizziness
EEG, EKG, and EMG changes
eye: irritation, miosis, tearing
extremities: aching, swelling, pain
GI irritation
hepatic damage
hyperthermia
hyporeflexia
hypotension
incontinence
mucous membrane irritation

muscle-twitching, tenderness,
   stiffness
myoglobinuria
nausea
neuritis
paralysis
paresthesia
peripheral neuropathy
respiratory: chest pain, cough,
   hyperpnea, rhinitis, respiratory
   depression
stupor
sweating
tachycardia
tremors
ulceration of mouth and throat
vasodilation
vomiting
weakness

Death due to peripheral vascular
   collapse

Chronic Exposure Effects

dermal: chloracne, dermatitis,
   depigmentation
paralysis

peripheral neuritis and neuropathy
porphyria

Suspected Effects

2,4-D:
   carcinogenesis 26
   demyelination and functional
      disturbances in the brain 8(III–
      114), 15(28)
   growth depression 22
   mutagenesis 22
   prenatal damage 1, 22, 23, 36

   Death due to ventricular
      fibrillation or cardiac
      failure, 1, 8(III–114)

MCPA:
   prenatal damage 11(264), 22, 23
   reproductive system effects 22
2,4,5-T:
   carcinogenesis 22
   prenatal damage 21(699), 23
2,4,5-TP:
   carcinogenesis 21(672), 22
   prenatal damage 21(672), 22

Toxicology
Chlorophenoxys depress the synthesis of RNase, uncouple oxidative phosphorylation, demyelinate nerves, and may produce hepatic peroxisomes. Skeletal muscle damage is manifest as myoglobinuria and creatinuria.

Additional Information
Chlorophenoxys have been contaminated with the dioxin 2,3,7,8-tetrachlorodibenzo-*p*-dioxin (TCDD). TCDD is a suspected teratogen, embryotoxin, carcinogen, and cocarcinogen, and may cause impaired cell-mediated immunity and aplastic anemia. In humans it has been associated with polyneuropathy, nystagmus, liver dysfunction, and enzyme imbalances leading to hirsutism, impotence, infertility, and chloracne 6(187–229). Controversy exists over its role in spontaneous abortions 6 (226). TCDD is a potent inducer of mixed function oxidases. It causes GI hemorrhage with necrosis and ulceration, cerebrovascular hemorrhage, hepatotoxicity, and atrophy of the lymphatic system 6(13,73).

2,4,5-T is commonly formulated with 2,4-D, dicamba, picloram, 2,4,5-TP, and MCPA.

Active Ingredients

acifluorfen	2,4-DB	MCPP
chlorophenoxyacetic acid	diclofop methyl	mecoprop (MCPP)
2,4-D	MCPA	2,4,5-T
	MCPB	2,4,5-TP

Copper Sulfate ────────────────────

Active Ingredient

Synonym: bordeaux powder
Use: algicide, fungicide, insecticide, molluscicide

Acute Exposure Effects

anemia
brain damage
capillary damage
CNS excitation followed by
  depression
coma
convulsions
copper in blood and urine
dermal: itching, discoloration
  (green), necrosis, dermatitis,
  keratinization of hands and feet
diarrhea
eye: irritation, edema,
  conjunctivitis, ulceration, and
  turbidity of cornea
fever
gastritis (hermorrhagic)
hair discoloration (green)
hemolysis
hepatic: centrilobular necrosis,
  hepatomegaly, jaundice, fatty
  liver, granuloma, fibrosis
hypotension
leukocytosis
metal fume fever

metallic taste
mucous membrane: irritation,
  burning, ulceration, congestion,
  atrophy, necrosis, perforation
muscle spasms
nausea
paralysis
pulse: weak
renal/urinary: fatty degeneration,
  tubular necrosis, anuria,
  azotemia, hemoglobinuria
respiratory: irritation, cough,
  burning sensation in chest and
  esophagus, sneezing
salivation
secretion of bile pigments
shock
sweating
tachycardia
tooth discoloration (green)
vomiting

Death due to hepatic, renal or
  circulatory failure, shock, coma,
  or convulsions

Chronic Exposure Effects

anorexia
chills
dermal: itching, necrosis dermatitis
eye: conjunctivitis, corneal
  ulceration and turbidity
fever
gastritis (hermorrhagic)

hepatic damage
hypersensitivity reaction
hypersusceptibility to infection
joint pain
metallic taste
mucous mebrane: irritation,
  necrosis, atrophy

Chronic Exposure Effects (*continued*)
muscle pain
respiratory: cough, dyspnea,
   pneumoconiosis with copper-
   containing nodules
rhinitis

rhinorrhagia
rhinorrhea
weakness
weight loss

Suspected Effects
carcinogenesis 7(57), 9(6), 27
hepatic: cirrhosis 7(57),
portal hypertension 7(57), 9(6)

mutagenesis 27
prenatal damage 27
pulmonary fibrosis 7(57)
reproductive system effects 27

Toxicology
Copper sulfate denatures proteins.

Additional Information
In blood, copper will be found in formed blood elements and not in serum. A type of chronic copper poisoning is recognized in the form of Wilson's disease (hereditary hepatolenticular degeneration).

Cyanides ————————————————————————

Class of Active Ingredients

Use: fumigants, insecticides, nematicides

Acute Exposure Effects

anxiety
aphasia
ascites
ataxia
blood: cherry red
brain anoxia
breath: bitter almond odor
burning sensation: mouth and
  tongue
cardiac arrhythmia
circulatory insufficiency
CNS depression
coma
confusion
convulsions
dermal: irritation, flushing, injury
dizziness
drowsiness
dysphagia
esophagus: mucosal erosion
eye: irritation, double vision,
  unreactive pupils, miosis/
  mydriasis
fever
giddiness
GI hyperemia
headache
hypertension followed by
  hypotension

mental depression
metallic taste
mucous membrane irritation
muscles: twitching, opisthotonus,
  trismus, sphincter control loss
myocardial weakness
nausea
palpitations
paralysis
paresis
psychotic behavior
pulse: irregular, weak
respiratory: irritation, pulmonary
  and laryngeal edema, depression,
  dyspnea, brochospasm, chest
  constriction, stertorus breathing,
  hyperpnea followed by
  bradypnea, pleural effusion
salivation
sweating
tachycardia followed by
  bradycardia
tremors
unconsciousness
vertigo
vomiting
weakness

Death due to respiratory failure

Chronic Exposure Effects
Same as above and in addition:

abdominal pain	hemorrhage	pulmonary edema
anemia	jaundice	thrombophlebitis
anorexia	leukocytosis	thyroid enlargement
cramps	mental deterioration	weight loss
dermatitis, hives	numbness	

Suspected Effects
  prenatal damage
    5(166)
Acrylonitrile:
  carcinogenesis 1,
    21(30), 28
  mutagenesis 21(31)

Toxicology
Cyanide pesticides are detoxified by conversion to the relatively harmless thiocyanate. Thiocyanate pesticides are partially metabolized to cyanide. Cyanide inactivates cytochrome oxidase and causes the cessation of cellular respiration. Effects are most noticeable on the brain and heart because of their greater oxygen consumption.

Active Ingredients

acrylonitrile
2- (2- butoxyethoxy) ethyl
  thiocyanate
calcium cyanide
cyanoethylene (acrylonitrile)

cyanogen chloride
hydrogen cyanide
isobornyl thiocyanoacetate
propenenitrile (acrylonitrile)
vinyl cyanide (acrylonitrile)

Cyclohexane ——————————————————

Inert Ingredient

Synonym: hexamethylene

Acute Exposure Effects

anesthesia
CNS depression
coma
cyclohexane in expired air, breath, blood, urine
cyclohexanone and cyclohexanol in blood
diarrhea
disequilibrium
excitement
eye: irritation, conjunctivitis
granulocytosis
hepatic damage
mucous membrane irritation

myocardial sensitization to epinepherine
narcosis
nausea
pneumonitis
renal damage
stupor
sulfonates and/or glucuronides in urine
unconsciousness
vomiting

Death due to respiratory failure

Chronic Exposure Effects
Chronic effects may occur, but no data were found.

Suspected Effects

diarrhea (chronic exposure) 3(3227)
glomerulonephritis 3(3227)
hepatocellular degeneration 3(3227), 14(137)

mutagenesis 27
vascular collapse leading to heart, lung, liver, and brain degeneration 14(137)

Toxicology
Cyclohexane is a fat solvent that causes CNS dysfunction and destruction of tissues. It is metabolized to cyclohexanone (see Cyclohexanone) and cyclohexanol, which enter the blood stream. These are conjugated with sulfonates or glucuronides prior to excretion.

Additional Information
Cyclohexane is frequently contaminated with benzene which may cause hematopoietic damage and leukemia (see Benzene).

For cyclohexane, there is a narrow margin between narcosis and death.

Persons with impaired pulmonary function may experience more severe symptoms and reflex bronchospasms.

Cyclohexanone

Inert Ingredient

Acute Exposure Effects
anxiety
CNS depression
dermal irritation
drowsiness
eye: irritation,
   conjunctivitis,
   transient corneal
   injury
mucous membrane
   irritation
narcosis
nausea
restlessness
vomiting
weight loss

Chronic Exposure Effects
corneal opacities
weight loss

Suspected Effects
bradycardia 3(4781)
bradypnea 3(4781)
cardiotoxicity 5(540)
hepatic damage 3(4781)
hypothermia 3(4780)
lymphocytosis/lymphocytopenia
   3(4781)
mutagenesis 27
neuromotor disturbances 3(4781)
oxygen consumption reduced
   3(4781)
paresis 3(4780)
postnatal damage 3(4780)
prenatal damage 3(4781)
renal damage 3(4781)

Toxicology
Cyclohexanone is a fat solvent that causes CNS dysfunction and the destruction of other tissues. It is reduced to cyclohexanol and conjugated with glucuronic acid.

Cycloheximide ⎯⎯⎯⎯⎯⎯⎯⎯⎯⎯⎯⎯⎯⎯⎯⎯

Active Ingredient

Use: fungicide

Exposure Effects

diarrhea	salivation
excitement	tremors
melena	

Suspected Effects
fatty liver 5(209)
mutagenesis 27
prenatal damage 26,
   27

Other effects may occur, but no data were found.

Toxicology
Cycloheximide inhibits protein synthesis.

Dalapon ———————————————————

Active Ingredient

Use: herbicide

Acute Exposure Effects

anorexia	eye: irritation,	lethargy
bradycardia	conjunctivitis,	respiratory tract
dermal irritation	corneal damage	irritation
diarrhea	GI disturbances	vomiting

Chronic Exposure Effects
Chronic effects may occur, but no data were found.

Suspected Effects
mutagenesis 27
renal damage 13
weight loss 13

Toxicology
Dalapon interferes with glucose utilization.

DEET

Active Ingredient

Synonyms: diethylbenzamide, diethyltoluamide
Use: repellent

Acute Exposure Effects
dermatitis

Other effects may exist, but no data were found.

Suspected Effects

aphasia 9(631)
aplastic anemia 9(631)
ataxia 9(631)
carcinogenesis 27
cardiac failure 9(630)
convulsions 9(630)
depression 9(630)
disorientation 9(631)
dorsiflexion of toes 9(631)
eye: irritation, tearing (bloody), conjunctivitis, corneal injury 9(630)
hypertrophy of liver, kidney, spleen, and testes 9(630)
jaundice 9(631)
mutagenesis 27
prenatal damage 9(631)
prostration 9(630)
respiratory failure 9(630)
stiffening into a sitting position 9(631)
tremors 9(630)

Toxicology
DEET is rapidly absorbed from the skin and distributed to all organs. It concentrates in brown fat, lacrimal glands, and the thyroid.

o-Dichlorobenzene

Active Ingredient

Use: insecticide

Acute Exposure Effects

CNS changes
dermal: irritation,
  blistering
drowsiness
erythropoesis
  depression

eye irritation
headache
hepatic damage
hyporeflexia
incoordination

mucous membrane
  irritation
nausea
neutropenia
renal damage
unconsciousness

Chronic Exposure Effects

anemia (hemolytic)
dermal: dermatitis
  (eczematoid), burns
exhaustion

eye: irritation, burns
gastric pain
headache

mucous membrane
  irritation (upper
  respiratory)
pallor
vomiting

Suspected Effects

anesthesia (general) 27
cholinesterase depression 3(3614)
CNS depression 3(3612)
leukemias (various) 3(3615), 9(165)
myelosis (proliferating) 3(3615)
peripheral leukoblastosis 3(3615)
pulmonary damage, pneumonitis
  3(3614), 14(258)

purpura 3(3615)
retroclavicular and peripheral
  lymphadenopathy 3(3615)
splenomegaly 3(3615)
urinary steroids elevated 3(3613)

p-Dichlorobenzene

Active Ingredient

> **Synonyms:** PDB, PDCB
> **Use:** insecticide

Acute Exposure Effects

ataxia
bradycardia
CNS depression
coma
convulusions
dermal: irritation, dermatitis
diarrhea
p-dichlorobenzene odor to urine
dizziness
drowsiness
eye: irritation, double vision, pain
headache
hepatic: jaundice, necrosis
mucous membrane irritation
muscle twitching
myocardial injury

nausea
renal damage
respiratory: laryngeal and
  pulmonary edema,
  bronchospasms, bradypnea
shock
tremor
unconsciousness
vomiting
weakness

Death due to pulmonary edema,
  respiratory failure, or ventricular
  fibrillation

Chronic Exposure Effects

anemia
ankle clonus
anorexia
dermal burns
erythrocytopenia

hemoglobinemia
hepatic: jaundice
hyperreflexia
methemoglobinemia

periorbital swelling
rhinitis
thrombocytopenia
weight loss

Suspected Effects

anemia (aplastic, hemolytic,
  hypochromic) 9(164)
ascites 3(3621)
cataracts 3(3622), 9(164)
dyspnea 3(3619), 9(164)
granulocytopenia 3(3619), 9(164)
hepatic: porphyria, hepatomegaly
  3(3619), cirrhosis 3(3621)
leukemia 3(3625)

mutagenesis 3(3625), 27
nystagmus 9(163)
oliguria 9(164)
paresthesia 3(3621)
petechial and purpurial rash 9(164)
pulmonary granulomatosis 3(3620)
renal: cloudy swelling 3(3619)
swelling of hands and feet 9(164)
tachypnea 3(3619), 9(163)

Toxicology

The metabolites 2,5-dichlorophenol and 2,5-dichloroquinol bind to hepatic proteins. The binding is proportional to the degree of liver necrosis.

Additional Information

There appear to be hyperreactive individuals. Fatalities have occurred following exposures to levels which cause no reaction in most individuals.

p-Dichlorobenzene may be contaminated with benzene (see Benzene).

Dichloroethyl Ether ━━━━━━━━━━━━━━━━━━━

Active Ingredient

Use: fumigant

Acute Exposure Effects
eye: irritation, tearing
mucous membrane irritation
nausea
respiratory: irritation, cough,
   pulmonary lesions, bronchitis

vomiting

Death due to respiratory
   collapse

Chronic Exposure Effects
bronchitis

Suspected Effects
brain congestion 3(2517)
carcinogenesis 1, 3(2518), 20, 27
dizziness 20
drowsiness 20
eye: conjunctivitis, corneal injury
   3(2518)

hepatic congestion 3(2517)
mutagenesis 27
pulmonary congestion 3(2517)
pulmonary edema 20
renal congestion 3(2517)
unconsciousness 20

Dimethyl Sulfoxide ———————————————————

Inert Ingredient

Synonyms: DMSO, methyl sulfoxide

Acute Exposure Effects

bronchopneumonia	eye irritation	lethary
chills	garlic odor to breath	nausea
cramps	hematuria	respiratory distress
dermal: irritation,	hepatic: jaundice	vomiting
urticarial wheals,		
burns		

Chronic Exposure Effects

Chronic effects may exist, but no data were found.

Suspected Effects

anaphylactic shock	corneal opacities	mutagenesis 27
18(614)	18(614)	prenatal damage
		5 (168), 26, 27

Toxicology

DMSO inhibits mixed function oxidases and produces reversible configurational changes in protein structure due to substitution of DMSO. It removes the lipid fraction of the stratum corneum, causing the release of histamine, holes, and shunts in the membrane, and alteration of the permeability of cell membranes and other membranes. Permeability changes lead to ionic shifts which are manifest, at the gross level, as blisters and swelling.

Additional Information

DMSO is synergistic with other toxicants because it facilitates penetration.

Dinitroanilines

Class of Active Ingredients

Use: fungicides, herbicides

Exposure Effects
dermal, eye, and mucous membrane irritation

Suspected Effects
Benefin:
  ataxia 23
  conjunctivitis 23
  edema 23
  erythema 23
  hyperactivity 23
Dicloran:
  carcinogenesis 22
  oculotoxicity 36(41)
Fluchloralin:
  bone marrow hyperplasia 23
  corneal opacities 23
  hemosiderosis 23
Isopropalin:
  carcinogenesis due to impurity *N*-nitroso-di-*n*-propylamine (NDPA) 31(79)
  corneal injury 31(86)

Penoxaline:
  hepatic lesions 23
  hepatomegaly 23
Profluralin:
  ataxia 23
  blood dyscrasias 23
  bradypnea 23
  carcinogenesis 23
  diarrhea 23
  ptosis 23
  salivation 23
Trifluralin:
  carcinogenesis 2(172), 23, 26 due to the impurity NDPA 22
  mutagenesis 22
  prenatal damage 22, 23

Toxicology
Dinitroanilines uncouple oxidative phosphorylation.

Active Ingredients

benefin	fluchloralin	pendimethalin
benfluralin	isopropalin	(penoxalin)
butralin	nitralin	penoxalin
dicloran	oryzalin	profluralin
dinitroamine		trifluralin

Dioxane —————————————————————————

Inert Ingredient

Acute Exposure Effects

abdominal pain
anorexia
coma
convulsions
dermal: drying,
　cracking
dizziness
drowsiness
eye: irritation, tearing
headache
hepatic damage

hypertension
leukocytosis
mucous membrane
　irritation
nausea
renal/urinary:
　albuminuria,
　glucosuria, HEAA
　in urine, renal
　damage, uremia

respiratory: irritation,
　coughing,
　pulmonary edema,
　congestion
vertigo
vomiting

Death due to kidney
　failure

Chronic Exposure Effects

cerebral edema
dermal: dermatitis,
　drying, cracking

eye irritation
headache
hepatic necrosis
nausea

renal/urinary: HEAA
　in urine, renal
　damage
respiratory irritation
vomiting

Suspected Effects

abdominal cramps (chronic
　exposure) 3(3952)
bladder distention 3(3948)
brain damage 3(3952), 25
BUN elevated 3(3952)
carcinogenesis 20, 25, 27, 28

mutagenesis 27
pneumonia 3(3952)
renal: enlargement 3(3948),
　obstruction 3(3950)
stomach: hemorrhagic areas in the
　pyloric region 3(3948)

Toxicology

Dioxane is a fat solvent that causes CNS dysfunction and the destruction of other tissues. It is partially metabolized to β-hydroxyethoxyacetic acid (HEAA).

Additional Information

Dioxane may form explosive peroxides during storage.

Diphenamid ─────────────────────────

Active Ingredient

Use: herbicide

Suspected Effects (reference 23)

ataxia	diarrhea	leukocytopenia
bradycardia	erythema	polyphagia
bradypnea	hemorrhage: oral,	polyuria
cardiomegaly	nasal, thymus	salivation
convulsions	hepatotoxicity	tearing
coughing	hyperthermia	thirst
depression	hypoactivity	vomiting

Endothall ———————————————————

Active Ingredient

Use: herbicide

Exposure Effects
dermal irritation
eye irritation
mucous membrane
   irritation

Suspected Effects
ataxia 15(79)
cardiac disorders 15(79)
circulatory disorders 15(79)
CNS disorders 15(79)
convulsions 15(79)
GI erosion and ulceration 15(79)
hematuria 27
respiratory depression 15(79)
shock 15(79)

Epichlorohydrin ─────────────────────────

Inert Ingredient

Synonym: chloromethyloxirane

Acute Exposure Effects
abdominal pain
CNS depression
cyanosis
dermal: irritation, sensitization
   blistering, burns, allergic
   eczematous contact dermatitis
eye irritation

hepatic damage
nausea
renal damage
respiratory: cough, irritation,
   pneumonitis (delayed onset),
   dyspnea, lung damage
vomiting

Chronic Exposure Effects
Chronic effects may exist, but no data were found.

Suspected Effects
carcinogenesis 20, 27
hepatic damage
   (chronic exposure)
   20

lung damage (chronic
   exposure) 20
mutagenesis 27
prenatal damage 26,
   27

pulmonary edema 27
renal damage (chronic
   exposure) 20
reproductive system
   damage 25, 27

Toxicology
Epichlorohydrin is a fat solvent that causes CNS dysfunction and destruction
of other tissues.

Ethyl Acetate ————————————————————

Inert Ingredient

Synonyms: acetic ester, acetic ether, ethyl ethanoate

Acute Exposure Effects

anemia
coma
dermatitis
dizziness
drowsiness
ethyl acetate in urine
eye: irritation, corneal
   lesions,
   conjunctivitis

headache
hepatic damage
leukocytopenia
mucous membrane
   irritation and
   damage
narcosis
nausea
renal damage

respiratory: irritation,
   pulmonary edema
unconsciousness
weakness

Chronic Exposure Effects

anemia
dermal: darkening,
   irritation
hepatomegaly

leukocytopenia
myocardial
   hypertrophy
renal hypertrophy

respiratory: bronchitis,
   pharyngitis, rhinitis
tooth erosion

Suspected Effects

carcinogenesis 27

Toxicology

Ethyl acetate is a fat solvent that causes CNS dysfunction and the destruction of other tissues.

Ethylene Oxide ────────────────────────────

Active and Inert Ingredient

> **Synonyms:** epoxyethane, ETO, oxirane
> **Use:** fumigant

Acute Exposure Effects

abdominal pain
anesthesia
bilirubinuria
bradycardia
CNS depression
coma
convulsions
cyanosis
dermal: dermatitis, injury
diarrhea
dizziness
drowsiness
eye: irritation, conjunctivitis,
　　corneal scarring, double vision,
　　tearing
headache

hepatic damage
mucous membrane irritation
nausea
renal damage
respiratory: dyspnea, hoarseness,
　　substernal pain, laryngeal and
　　pulmonary edema,
　　bronchospasm, respiratory
　　depression, coughing of frothy
　　sputum
tremor
vomiting
weakness

Death due to pulmonary edema or
　　respiratory failure

Chronic Exposure Effects

bilirubinuria
hematopoietic system
　　damage

hepatic damage
renal damage
testicular damage

Suspected Effects

carcinogenesis 20, 27
mutagenesis 20, 22, 27
postnatal damage 27

prenatal damage 27
reproductive system
　　damage 22, 27

Toxicology
Ethylene oxide is a fat solvent that causes CNS dysfunction and tissue destruction. It behaves as a cytotoxic alkylating agent, causing denaturation and precipitation of proteins.

Ethyl Formate

Active Ingredient

Use: fumigant

Acute Exposure Effects

abdominal pain
CNS depression
convulsions
cyanosis
dermatitis
diarrhea
dizziness
drowsiness
eye: irritation, conjunctivitis,
  tearing, double vision,
mucous membrane irritation
narcosis
nasusea

respiratory: irritation, hoarseness,
  substernal pressure, chest pain,
  dyspnea, laryngeal edema,
  bronchospasm, pulmonary
  edema, respiratory depression,
  coughing of frothy sputum
tremor
unconsciousness
vomiting

Death due to pulmonary edema,
  respiratory failure, or circulatory
  failure

Chronic Exposure Effects
Chronic effects may exist, but no data were found.

Suspected Effects
carcinogenesis 26, 27

Toxicology
Ethyl formate is a defatting agent.

Eugenol

Active and Inert Ingredient

Use: attractant

Acute Exposure Effects

anemia
coma
CNS depression
dermal: irritation, inflammatory infiltrates
gastroenteritis and excess mucin secretion

hematuria
hypotension
lethargy
localized anesthesias
mucous membrane irritation
muscle relaxation
prostration

pulmonary edema
residues of bromide in tissue
vomiting

Death due to peripheral vascular collapse

Chronic Exposure Effects
Chronic effects may exist, but no data were found.

Suspected Effects

adrenal hypertrophy 3(2534)
corneal opacities 23
dermal: erythema, ulcers 3(2534); keratosis 3(2534)
hepatomegaly 3(2534)
hyperplasia 3(2534)
motor incoordination 3(2534)
mutagenesis 27
myocardial contractile force decreased 3(2534)

osteoporosis 3(2534)
paralysis 17(1692)
renal damage manifest by urinary incontinence 17(1692)
stomach: desquamation of epithelium, punctate hemorrhages in pyloric and glandular regions 3(2534)

Toxicology
Eugenol inhibits the oxidation of flavin-linked and NAD-linked substrates. It causes the denaturation of cytoplasmic proteins, loss of staining capacity of the epithelium, loss of cell boundaries, cellular swelling, and cell necrosis.

Formaldehyde ─────────────────────────────

Active and Inert Ingredient

Use: fumigant, inert ingredient

Acute Exposure Effects

abdominal pain
anesthesia
anxiety
burning sensation in nose and
  throat
clammy skin
CNS depression
coma
convulsions
cyanosis
dermal: coagulation necrosis,
  dermatitis, hypersensitivity
diarrhea
dizziness
dysphagia
eye: tearing, burns, double vision,
  conjunctivitis
GI irritation and necrosis
headache
hematemesis
hoarseness
metabolic acidosis
mucous membrane irritation

nausea
pallor
renal/urinary: renal injury, dysuria,
  anuria, pyuria, formate in urine,
  hematuria
respiratory: pneumonia, dyspnea,
  wheezing, pulmonary edema,
  laryngeal edema, bronchospasm,
  respiratory depression, coughing
  of frothy fluid, obstructive
  tracheobronchitis, laryngeal
  spasms, substernal pressure
shock
stupor
thirst
unconsciousness
vertigo
vomiting
weakness

Death due to pulmonary edema,
  respiratory failure, or circulatory
  collapse

Chronic Exposure Effects

bronchitis
cough
dermal: dermatitis
  and sensitization

formate in urine
vital capacity reduced

Suspected Effects

carcinogenesis
  3(2645), 20, 27, 28
mutagenesis 20, 27

postnatal damage 27
prenatal damage 27

reproductive system
  damage 27

Toxicology

Formaldehyde reacts with the mucosa of the alimentary and respiratory tracts, combining with functional groups and initiating polymerization reactions. It is rapidly oxidized to formic acid in most tissues. The resulting acidosis, lactic acidemia, and decreased circulation may be responsible for CNS disturbances. Formaldehyde can react with hydrochloric acid in the stomach to produce bis-chloromethyl ether, which is carcinogenic to humans.

Additional Information

Susceptibility of the mucous membranes to formaldehyde decreases with repeated exposures. However, in some individuals, sensitization to inhalation exposure has occurred.

Formamidines

Class of Active Ingredients

Use: acaricides, fungicides, insecticides

Acute Exposure Effects

abdominal pain
anorexia
back pain
fever
heat sensitivity

neuromuscular
  disorders
prostaglandin
  depression
rash on arms and face
sweet taste

urinary: bladder
  irritation,
  hematuria,
  hemorrhagic
  cystitis, proteinuria
vomiting

Chronic Exposure Effects

bladder irritation
heat intolerance
muscle relaxation

rash on arms and face
sleepiness
urinary abnormalities

Suspected Effects

Amitraz:

carcirogenesis 22
mutagenesis 22

Chlordimeform:

anemia 22
bile duct hyperplasia and
  pericholangitis 36
blood dyscrasias 22
carcinogenesis 22
convulsions 36
hepatic nodules and focal
  hyperplasia 36
humoral immune response
  suppression 37
hyperactivity 36
leukocytosis 22
methemoglobinemia 22
mutagenesis 22
renal pigmentation 22
respiratory arrest 36
postnatal damage 36
prenatal damage 22
tremors 36
weight depression 22

Toxicology
Formamidines block neuromuscular transmission, inhibit monoamine oxidase, uncouple oxidative phosphorylation, inhibit prostaglandin biosynthesis, and induce accumulation of serotonin and norepinephrine in the brain.

Additional Information
Chlordimeform is often formulated with toxaphene and methyl parathion.

Active Ingredients

amitraz
chlordimeform

chlorophenamidine
 (chlordimeform)
formetanate

Glycerol Formal _____

Inert Ingredient

Acute Exposure Effects

anemia	fever	nausea
coma	glycerol in urine	paralysis
convulsions	hematuria	pneumonitis
diarrhea	mucous membrane	restlessness
eye irritation	irritation	vomiting

Chronic Exposure Effects
Chronic effects may exist, but no data were found.

Suspected Effects
Prenatal damage 27

Halocarbon Fumigants ⎯⎯⎯⎯⎯⎯⎯⎯⎯⎯⎯

Class of Active and Inert Ingredients

Use: fungicides, insecticides, nematicides, and rodenticides

Acute Exposure Effects
anesthesias
anorexia
ataxia
behavioral disorders
CNS depression
coma
confusion
convulsions
dermal: dermatitis, burns
dizziness
eye: tearing, burns, conjunctivitis,
   double vision
giddiness
headache
hepatic: jaundice, necrosis,
   hepatomegaly, fatty infiltration;
   elevated serum alkaline
   phosphatase, bilirubin, GOT,
   GPT, and LDH
hyporeflexia
mucous membrane irritation

muscle twitching
myocardial injury
nausea
renal/urinary: anuria/oliguria,
   proteinuria, tubular necrosis,
   glycosuria; elevated BUN, NPN,
   and creatinine
respiratory: bronchospasm,
   bradypnea, depression,
   pulmonary and laryngeal edema
shock
tremors
unconsciousness
vertigo
vomiting
weakness

Death due to CNS depression, renal
   failure, pulmonary edema,
   respiratory failure, ventricular
   fibrillation, circulatory collapse

Chronic Exposure Effects
All of the Above Plus:
paralysis
paresthesia
increased
   susceptibility to
   viral hepatitis

Additional Exposure Effects of Individual Halocarbon Fumigants

Carbon Tetrachloride:
  abdominal pain
  aplastic anemia
  dehydration
  diarrhea
  drowsiness
  edema
  eye: amblyopia, loss of peripheral
    color perception, scotomata
  hematemesis
  hemoglobinuria
  hypothrombinemia
  leukocyturia
  memory loss
  Parkinsonism
  polyneuritis

Chloroform:
  abdominal pain
  diarrhea
  dyspnea
  hypothrombinemia

Chloropicrin:
  diarrhea
  methemoglobinemia
  muscle necrosis
  orthostatic hypotension
  respiratory: cough with frothy
    sputum, pulmonary congestion,
    pulmonary hemorrhage,
    wheezing, bronchitis

Dibromochloropropane:
  male sterility
  testicular atrophy

1,3-Dichloropropene:
  abdominal pain
  chest discomfort
  coughing of frothy sputum
  dyspnea
  irritability
  memory loss

Ethylene Dibromide:
  abdominal pain
  anemia
  dermal sensitization
  diarrhea
  fertility decreased
  insomnia
  pallor
  restlessness
  tachycardia
  urine: dark

Ethylene Dichloride:
  abdominal pain
  adrenal damage
  anemia
  collapse
  cyanosis
  diarrhea
  dyspnea
  epigastric cramps
  hemorrhage
  hyperemia
  hypotension
  pallor

Methyl Bromide:
  abdominal pain
  aphasia
  areflexia
  ataxia
  collapse
  cyanosis
  delirium
  encephalopathy
  eye: blurred vision, strabismus,
    temporary blindness
  itching
  muscle pain
  pallor
  respiratory: coughing of frothy
    sputum, dyspnea, pneumonitis,
    tachypnea
  status epilepticus

Death due to circulatory or
  respiratory collapse

Additional Exposure Effects of Individual Halocarbon Fumigants (*continued*)

Methylene Chloride:
  carboxyhemoglobin levels elevated
  irritability
  pneumonia
  splenic atrophy
Propylene Dichloride:
  coughing of frothy sputum
  dyspnea
  irritability
  memory loss

1,1,1-Trichloroethane:
  sensitization of the heart to
    epinephrine
Trichloroethylene:
  hallucinations
  sleep pattern changes

Suspected Effects

Carbon Tetrachloride:
  adrenal damage 12(386)
  carcinogenesis 12(388), 20, 28
  postnatal damage 27
  prenatal damage 1, 12(384), 27
  reproductive system effects 12(384),
    27
Chloroform:
  carcinogenesis 12(417), 20, 28
  prenatal damage 27
  reproductive system effects 27
Chloropicrin:
  carcinogenesis 26
  hemosiderosis 23
Dibromochloropropane:
  carcinogenesis 12(91), 20, 22, 28
  mutagenesis 12(91), 22, 27
  prenatal damage 27
  reproductive system effects 22, 27
1,3-Dichloropropene:
  mutagenesis 20, 27
Ethylene Dibromide:
  carcinogenesis 3(3501), 20, 25, 28
  mutagenesis 3(3500), 22, 25
  postnatal damage 4(A-64), 25
  prenatal damage 4(A-64), 22, 25, 27
  reproductive system effects 3(3500),
    4(A-64), 22, 27
Ethylene Dichloride:
  carcinogenesis 12(442), 20, 27, 28
  mutagenesis 27

Methyl Bromide:
  carcinogenesis 20
  diarrhea 22
  mutagenesis 27
  paralysis 22
  polyuria 22
  prenatal damage 22
  reproductive system effects 22
  salivation 22
  thirst 22
Methylene Chloride:
  carcinogenesis 20, 27
  mutagenesis 27
  postnatal damage 27
  prenatal damage 27
Perchloroethylene:
  carcinogenesis 1, 12(505) 20(638),
    27
  hematuria 1
  postnatal damage 27
  prenatal damage 1, 27
Propylene Dichloride:
  adrenal injury 3(3530)
  mutagenesis 3(3532), 27
1,1,1,-Trichloroethane:
  carcinogenesis 12(525)
  mutagenesis 27
  prenatal damage 27
Trichloroethylene:
  carcinogenesis 12(561), 27
  mutagenesis 12(561), 27
  prenatal damage 27
  reproductive system effects 27

Toxicology

Halocarbon fumigants inhibit several enzyme systems, including the sulfhydryl enzymes and hexokinases. They are alkylating agents that may react with protein and DNA. They are also fat solvents that attack the methylene bridges of unsaturated fatty acids, causing skin and mucous membrane damage. Neurotoxic effects may be delayed hours or days.

Carbon tetrachloride is readily metabolized to a free radical that causes lipid peroxidation and consequent damage to the liver, lungs, kidneys, testes, and adrenals. It binds to, and may destroy, cytochrome P-450 in liver microsomes.

Chloroform reacts with cardiac protein. It interferes with the microsomal enzyme system.

Dibromochloropropane causes a reduction in the metabolism of glucose to carbon dioxide in sperm, leading to infertility. It causes seminiferous tubular degeneration, resulting in testicular atrophy in animals.

Ethylene dibromide may be carcinogenic due to the properties of its metabolite bromoacetaldehyde.

Methylene chloride is metabolized in part to carbon monoxide.

Additional Information

The neurotoxic effects of halocarbon fumigants may be delayed for hours or days. They readily penetrate skin, protective gear, and respirator adsorbents. Cooking may volatilize residues in food. Groups with special susceptibilities include the following:

> cardiac patients
> persons exposed to alcohol
> persons with anemia (methylene chloride only)
> persons exposed to carbon monoxide (methylene chloride only)

Ethylene dichloride can produce phosgene gas under conditions of incomplete combustion.

Active and Inert Ingredients

1,2-bromoethane (ethylene dibromide)	active ingredient
bromomethane (methyl bromide)	active ingredient
carbon dichloride (perchloroethylene)	active and inert ingredient
carbon tetrachloride	active and inert ingredient
chlorallylchloride (1,3-dichloropropene)	active ingredient
chloroethane (1,1,1-trichloroethane)	active and inert ingredient
chloroform	active and inert ingredient
chloropicrin	active ingredient
DBCP (dibromochloropropane)	active ingredient
DD®	active ingredient

Active and Inert Ingredients (*continued*)

dibromochloropropane	active ingredient
1,2-dibromoethane (ethylene dibromide)	active ingredient
1,2-dichloroethane (ethylene dichloride)	active and inert ingredient
dichloromethane (methylene chloride)	active and inert ingredient
1,2-dichloropropane (propylene dichloride)	active and inert ingredient
1,3-dichloropropene	active and inert ingredient
EDB (ethylene dibromide)	active ingredient
EDC (ethylene dichloride)	active and inert ingredient
ethylene dibromide	active ingredient
ethylene dichloride	active and inert ingredient
ethylene trichloride (trichloroethylene)	active and inert ingredient
methyl bromide	active ingredient
methyl chloroform (1,1,1,-trichloroethane)	active and inert ingredient
methylene chloride	active and inert ingredient
methylene dichloride (methylene chloride)	active and inert ingredient
monobromomethane (methyl bromide)	active ingredient
nitrochloroform (chloropicrin)	active ingredient
perchloroethylene	active and inert ingredient
perchloromethane (carbon tetrachloride)	active and inert ingredient
propylene dichloride	active and inert ingredient
tetrachloroethylene (perchloroethylene)	active and inert ingredient
tetrachloromethane (carbon tetrachloride)	active and inert ingredient
1,1,1-trichloroethane	active and inert ingredient
trichloroethene (trichloroethylene)	active and inert ingredient
trichloroethylene	active and inert ingredient
trichloromethane (chloroform)	active and inert ingredient
trichloronitromethane (chloropicrin)	active ingredient

Hexachlorobenzene _____

Active Ingredient

Synonym: perchlorobenzene
Use: fungicide

Acute Exposure Effects
See Pentachlorophenol for additional effects.

dermal irritation
drowsiness
incoordination

mucous membrane
  irritation
unconsciousness

Chronic Exposure Effects
See Pentachlorophenol for additional effects.

abdominal pain
anorexia/weight loss
arthritis (painless)
atrophy of hands, muscles, and skin
corneal opacity
dermal: dermatitis,
  photosensitivity, alopecia/
  hirsutism, sclerodermoid
  thickening, scarring of hands and
  face, hyperpigmentation,
  rhagades, fragile skin, burns

digit deformation and shortening
hepatic damage
hypothermia
paresthesias
porphyria
thyroid enlargement
urine: port wine color

Suspected Effects
anemia 3(3634), 9(588)
ataxia 3(3629)
bone marrow effects 36
carcinogenesis 3(3643), 12(168), 27,
  28
convulsions 9(588)
fibrosis of lungs and heart 9(593)
hypocalcemia 3(3634)
hypoglycemia 3(3634)
immunotoxicity 3(3644)
irritability 3(3629)
lung damage 14(258)

mutagenesis 27
neurotoxicity 3(3628)
oliguria 9(588)
paralysis 3(3629), 9(588)
postnatal damage 4(A–18), 9(592),
  27
prenatal damage 4(A–18), 9(592),
  12(166), 27
reproductive system effect 9(592)
tremor 3(3629), 9(588)
renal damage 14(258)

Toxicology
Pentachlorophenol is the primary metabolite (see Pentachlorophenol). Hexachlorobenzene interferes with lipid metabolism and transport. It also induces liver microsomal enzymes.

Hexachlorophene ─────────────────────────────

Active Ingredient

Use: bactericide, fungicide

Acute Exposure Effects

cardiomyopathy	diarrhea	temperature
circulatory failure	headache	fluctuations
CNS lesions	prenatal damage	twitching
convulsions	shock	

Suspected Effects
carcinogenesis 26, 27
postnatal damage 27
reproductive system
   effects 22

Additional Information
TCDD is a possible impurity (see Chlorophenoxys for more information on TCDD).

Isophorone —————————————————————

Inert Ingredient

Acute Exposure Effects

CNS disturbances
dermal irritation
dizziness
eye: irritation,
   conjunctivitis
faintness
fatigue

feeling of suffocation
headache
inebriation
malaise
mucous membrane
   irritation
narcosis

nausea
pneumonitis
respiratory distress

Death due to narcosis
   (CNS depression) or
   irritation of the lungs

Chronic Exposure Effects
Chronic effects may occur, but no data were found.

Suspected Effects

corneal necrosis and
   opacities 18(753)
renal damage 18(753)

Toxicology
Isophorone is metabolized via methyl group oxidation and conjugated with glucuronic acid.

Kerosene —————————————————————————

Active and Inert Ingredient

> **Composition:** dinuclear aromatics 5%, branched paraffins 11%, tricyclo paraffins 1%, dicyclo paraffins 12%, mononuclear aromatics 16%, paraffins 25%, monocyclo paraffins 30%
> **Use:** insecticide

Acute Exposure Effects

anemia (aplastic)
anorexia
aphasia
ataxia
burning sensation in mouth, chest, esophagus, and stomach
cardiac dilation
chills
CNS depression
collapse
coma
confusion
convulsions
cyanosis
depression/euphoria
dermal: irritation, dermatitis, blistering, edema, infection, and defatting
diarrhea (bloody)
disorientation
distress
dizziness
drowsiness/insomnia
eye: irritation, conjunctivitis, vision blurred
fatigue
fever
GI upset
headache
hemoglobinemia
hepatic: jaundice, hepatomegaly

hypertension
insomnia
kerosene in blood and expired air
leukocytosis
mucous membrane irritation
nausea
nervousness
neutropenia
pallor
paresthesias
positive Romberg sign
renal injury
respiratory: irritation, tachypnea, bronchopneumonia, chest pain, pulmonary edema and lesions, dyspnea, cough, hemorrhage, rales, pneumonitis
rhinorrhagia
splenomegaly
sweating
tachycardia
tinnitus
twitching
urine: cells, casts, albumin
vomiting
weakness

Death due to hemorrhagic pulmonary edema, bronchopneumonia, renal dysfunction, fibrillation, respiratory arrest, and cardiac failure

Chronic Exposure Effects

albuminuria	dizziness	pain in limbs
anemia (aplastic)	leukocytosis	paresthesia
bone marrow	nervousness	weakness
suppression and	neutropenia	weight loss
hypoplasia	numbness	

Suspected Effects

bladder congestion 24(105)
blood glucose depression 24(106)
hepatic: vacuolation 24(104),
  hyperemia 24(105)
mental depression 24(61)

pneumonia (chronic) 24(112)
renal: cloudy degeneration of renal
  tubules, glomeruli and pelves
  congestion 24(104)

Toxicology
Kerosene is a fat solvent that causes CNS dysfunction and damage to other tissues. In cases of acute exposure, severe liver damage is the primary toxic effect, which may lead to a decrease in blood glucose levels and result in coma or convulsions and death. Kerosene inhibits protein synthesis.

Additional Information
Kerosene may be contaminated with benzene (see Benzene).

Maleic Anhydride ————————————————

Inert Ingredient

Acute Exposure Effects

asthmatic reaction
dermal: irritation, burns
diarrhea
dizziness
drowsiness
erythrocytosis
eye: irritation, double vision,
   photophobia, conjunctivitis,
   corneal erosion, and burns
fatigue
headache

hematocrit increased
hypotension
mucous membrane irritation
nausea
respiratory: irritation, coughing,
   dyspnea, pulmonary edema,
   sneezing
rhinorrhagia
vomiting
weakness

Chronic Exposure Effects

allergic sensitization
asthmatic reaction
bronchitis

chronic cough
dermatitis
GI disturbances

Suspected Effects

carcinogenesis 27
pulmonary edema
   (chronic exposure)
   20

Additional Information
Maleic anhydride emits toxic fumes when heated.

Maleic Hydrazide ────────────────────────

Active Ingredient

Use: growth regulator, herbicide

Suspected Effects
carcinogenesis 22, 26,
   27, 36
mutagenesis 22, 27
postnatal damage 36

Other effects may occur, but no data were found.

Mercurials (Inorganic and Organic) ⸻

Class of Active Ingredients

Use: fungicides

Acute Exposure Effects

abdominal pain
acidosis
agitation
anesthesia
anxiety
apathy
ataxia
CNS injury
collapse
coma
convulsions
deafness
delirium with hallucinations
dermal: burns, dermatitis,
    sensitization
diarrhea: bloody
dysphasia
edema: generalized
eye: field constriction, blindness,
    ulceration of the cornea and
    conjunctiva
emotional instability
fatigue
GI: gastroenteritis, ulceration,
    hemmorrhage
headache
hepatic necrosis
hypercholesterolemia
jaw: movement difficult, necrosis
manic-depressive psychosis

memory loss
metallic taste
mucous membrane irritation
muscle weakness
nausea
pallor
paralysis
paresis
paresthesias
prostration
pulse: weak
renal/urinary: nephrosis, polyuria/
    anuria, tubular necrosis,
    albuminuria, azotemia,
    cylindruria, hematuria
respiratory: bronchitis, hypopnea,
    bronchiolitis, pneumonitis
salivation
stomatitis
tachycardia
tenesmus
thirst
throat pain
tremors: finger, eyelid, tongue
vomiting: bloody, electrolyte loss
weight loss

Death due to peripheral vascular
    collapse or renal failure

Chronic Exposure Effects

anorexia/weight loss
anxiety
aphasia
ataxia
coma

deafness
delirium with hallucinations
dermal: dermatitis, edema, papules,
    ulcers, sensitization
diarrhea

Chronic Exposure Effects (*continued*)

dysphagia
encephalopathy
eye: lens opacities, tunnel vision,
    blindness
excitability
fatigue
gums: gingivitis, black line
indigestion
insomnia
irritability
manic-depressive psychosis
memory loss
metallic taste
mouth ulceration

muscular weakness
neurologic damage
paralysis
paresthesia
postnatal damage
prenatal damage
renal/urinary: tubular necrosis,
    albuminuria, azotemia,
    hematuria
salivation
teeth loosening
tremors: hands, feet, tongue, lips,
    eyelids, fingers

Suspected Effects

carcinogenesis 27

Toxicology

Inorganic and organic forms of mercury produce similar signs and symptoms with the organic forms being faster acting.

Mercurials:
—bind to neural membranes and accumulate in the brain;
—bind to purines in DNA;
—are zinc antimetabolites;
—inhibit the hepatic microsomal detoxification system, thus increasing the toxicity of other toxins;
—bind to phosphoryl and sulfhydryl groups, thereby changing cell membrane permeability and macromolecular conformation.

Active Ingredients

bismethyl mercuric sulfate
Ceresan®
ethylmercuriothio salicylate
ethyl mercury
mercuric chloride
mercuriothiolate (ethylmercuriothio
    salicylate)
mercurous chloride

2-methoxyethyl mercuric chloride
methyl mercury
phenyl mercury acetate
PMA (phenyl mercury acetate)
thimersal (ethylmercuriothio
    salicylate)
thiomerosalate (ethylmercuriothio
    salicylate)

Metalaxyl _____

Active Ingredient

Use: fungicide

Suspected Effects
conjunctivitis 32(65)
corneal opacity 32(65)
elevated alkaline
   phosphatase 32(59)

Other effects may occur, but no data were found.

Metaldehyde ———————————————————

Active Ingredient

Use: molluscicide

Acute Exposure Effects

abdominal pain
asthmatic attack
ataxia
coma
convulsions
depression
diarrhea
drowsiness
dyspnea
fever
flushing

hepatic damage
hypertension
incontinence
nausea
opisthotonus
renal/urinary: renal
   damage,
   albuminuria,
   urinary casts,
   aciduria
rhinorrhea

risus sardonicus
salivation
sweating
tachycardia followed
   by bradycardia
tearing
unconsciousness
vomiting

Death due to renal
   failure or respiratory
   failure

Chronic Exposure Effects
Chronic effects may occur, but no data were found.

Suspected Effects
mutagenesis 27
postnatal damage 27
reproductive system
   damage 27

Toxicology
Metaldehyde is metabolized to acetaldehyde. Metaldehyde is parasym-
pathomimetic.

Methyl Formate ————————————————

Active Ingredient

Use: fumigant

Acute Exposure Effects

abdominal pain
anesthesia
CNS depression
convulsions
cyanosis
dermatitis
diarrhea
dizziness
eye: irritation, temporary blindness,
  conjunctivitis, double vision,
  tearing
headache
mucous membrane irritation
narcosis

nausea
respiratory: substernal pressure,
  hoarseness, chest pain, laryngeal
  and pulmonary edema,
  respiratory depression, dyspnea,
  coughing of frothy fluid
tremor
unconsciousness
vomiting
weakness

Death due to pulmonary edema or
  respiratory failure

Chronic Exposure Effects
Chronic effects may occur, but no data were found.

Suspected Effects
ataxia 1

Methyl Ketones ─────────────────────────────

Class of Inert Ingredients

Acute Exposure Effects

coma

conjugated glucuronic acid in urine

CNS and peripheral neuropathy

dermatitis

dizziness

drowsiness

eye irritation

GI disturbances

headache

mucous membrane irritation

narcosis

paresthesias

respiratory: distress, pulmonary
  edema

vomiting

weakness

Death due to CNS depression

Chronic Exposure Effects

abdominal distress

anorexia

CNS disturbances

dermatitis

eye irritation

headache

nausea

Additional Effects of Individual Methyl Ketones

Methyl n-butyl Ketone:

distal neuropathy

Methyl Isobutyl Ketone:

colitis

heartburn

hepatomegaly

somnolence/insomia

Suspected Effects

Methyl Isobutyl Ketone:

renal proximal tubular damage and
  enlargement 1

Toxicology

Methyl *n*-butyl ketone is metabolized to 2,5-hexanedione, a neurotoxin, which causes thinning of myelin and axonal swelling. This causes peripheral neuropathies and CNS damage.

Active and Inert Ingredients

methyl *n*-amyl ketone	inert ingredient
methyl *n*-butyl ketone	inert ingredient
methyl ethyl ketone	inert ingredient
methyl isoamyl ketone	inert ingredient
methyl isobutyl ketone	inert ingredient
methyl nonyl ketone	active ingredient
methyl propyl ketone	inert ingredient

Methyl Methacrylate (Monomer) ────────────

Inert Ingredient

Acute Exposure Effects
anorexia	eye irritation	mucous membrane
cardiac arrest	excitement/narcosis	irritation
dermatitis	hypotension	unconsciousness
drowsiness		

Chronic Exposure Effects
Chronic effects may exist, but no data were found.

Suspected Effects
carcinogenesis 27

mutagenesis 27

prenatal damage
   5(547), 27

reproductive system
   damage 27

Additional Information
Methyl methacrylate is especially dangerous to elderly individuals.

Mineral Spirits ────────────────────

Inert Ingredient

> **Composition:** 1% olefins, 13–19% aromatics, 80–86% saturated hydrocarbons

Acute Exposure Effects

anemia
cardiac arrhythmia
CNS disturbances
coma
convulsions
dermatitis
eye irritation
fatigue
GI irritation

headache
hematuria
mucous membrane
   irritation
nausea
respiratory: irritation,
   coughing, bronchial
   pneumonia, and
   depression

unconsciousness
vomiting
weakness
weight loss

Death due to respiratory
   failure

Chronic Exposure Effects

anemia
dizziness
hematuria

nervousness
pain in limbs
paresthesia

proteinuria
weakness
weight loss

Suspected Effects

hepatic: focal necrosis 24(92–93)
respiratory: pulmonary congestion,
   inflammatory infiltrates 24(92),
   emphysema 24(93)

Toxicology

Mineral spirits are fat solvents that cause CNS dysfunction and destruction of other tissues.

Additional Information

May contain benzene (see Benzene).

Naphthalenes ————————————————————

Class of Active Ingredients

Use: fumigants, rodent repellents

Acute Exposure Effects

abdominal pain and disorders
allergic sensitization
anemia (hemolytic)
anorexia
CNS depression
coma
confusion
convulsions
dermal: dermatitis,
    photosensitivity, facial flushing
diarrhea
dizziness
drowsiness/excitement
eye: blindness, double vision,
    corneal ulceration, cataracts,
    optic neuritis
headache
hyperthermia
jaundice
leukocytosis
methemoglobinemia
mucous membrane irritation
nausea

pallor
red blood cells: Heinz bodies,
    nucleation, hematocrit and
    hemoglobin depression
renal/urinary: tubular blockage,
    azotemia, albuminuria, bladder
    irritation, dysuria, anuria/
    oliguria, presence of metabolites
    α- and β-naphthol and
    naphthquinone in urine,
    discolored urine, odor of
    naphthalene in urine, hematuria,
    hemoglobinuria
respiratory: bronchospasm,
    laryngeal edema, depression
sweating
vomiting
weakness
tremor

Death due to respiratory or renal
    failure

Chronic Exposure Effects

anemia
anorexia
coma
convulsions
dermatitis
diarrhea
dizziness
eye: corneal ulcers, cataracts, optic
    neuritis
headache
hepatic injury

kernicterus
leukocytosis
nausea
pallor
red blood cells: Heinz bodies,
    nucleation, hematocrit and
    hemoglobin depression
renal/urinary: renal injury, dysuria,
    hematuria, odor of naphthalene
    in urine, discolored urine
sweating

Suspected Effects

ataxia 34(32)

dyspnea 34(32)

jaundice (delayed) in infants
    exposed during pregnancy 9(136)

prenatal damage 9(136)

prostration 34(32)

Toxicology

Naphthalenes are metabolized by the cytochrome P-450 system. The metabolites, and not the parent compound, are toxic.

Additional Information

Persons with a glucose-6-phosphate dehydrogenase deficiency may be hypersusceptible to naphthalene poisoning.

Vapor from moth balls or items stored with them may cause symptoms. Infants are especially sensitive, and fatal kernicterus has been caused by naphthalene moth ball treated materials.

Active Ingredients

NAA (naphthalene acetic acid)

naphthalene

napthalene acetic acid

1,8-naphthalic anhydride

naphthylacetic acid (naphthalene
    acetic acid)

tar camphor (naphthalene)

Nicotines ─────────────────────────────

Class of Active Ingredients

Use: insecticides

Acute Exposure Effects

abdominal pain
anorexia
ataxia
auditory disturbances
blood: elevation of glucose, fatty
　acids, potassemia
bradycardia followed by
　tachycardia
cardiac arrhythmia
CNS and peripheral nervous system
　stimulation followed by
　depression
coma
confusion
convulsions (clonic)
cyanosis
dermal irritation
diarrhea
dizziness
EEG and EKG abnormalities
endocrine stimulation
eye: irritation, miosis/mydriasis,
　vision disturbed
GI disturbance
headache
hemorrhage (internal)
hyperemia
hyperperistalsis

hypertension followed by
　hypotension
hyperthermia
insomnia
muscle twitching and weakness
nausea
paralysis
phagocytosis impaired
prostration
pulse: irregular
renal/urinary: renal injury, cotinine
　and isomethonium in urine,
　polyuria/oliguria, glycosuria
respiratory: cough, dyspnea,
　sneezing, substernal pressure,
　tachypnea, followed by
　respiratory paralysis
salivation
sweating
tremors
vasoconstriction followed by
　vasodilation
vomiting
weakness

Death due to respiratory paralysis,
　convulsions, or circulatory and
　renal failure

Chronic Exposure Effects

cardiac rhythm
　disturbance
GI disturbance

vasoconstriction
visual disturbance

Suspected Effects

carcinogenesis 20
cocarcinogenesis 20
prenatal damage
  3(2744), 4(A–82),
  20

reproductive system
  effects 3(2744)

Toxicology

Nicotines:

—stimulate nicotinic receptors in the sympathetic and parasympathetic postganglionic neurons and the skeletal muscle fibers at the neuromuscular junction;

—mimic acetylcholine, thereby causing initial excitation at acetylcholine receptors followed by depression and paralysis;

—are metabolized fairly quickly to less toxic compounds.

Active Ingredients

anabasine
neonicotine
  (anabasine)

nicotine
nornicotine

Nitrophenols ―――――――――――――――――――

Class of Active Ingredients

Use: acaricides, fungicides, herbicides, insecticides

Acute Exposure Effects

abdominal pain
acidosis
agranulocytosis
anorexia
basal metabolic rate elevated
cerebral edema
CNS stimualtion followed by
   depression
collapse
coma
convulsions
cyanosis
dehydration
dermal: dermatitis, flushing, yellow
   staining
diarrhea
dizziness
excitement
GI upset
hair: yellow staining
headache
heat sensitivity/stroke
hepatic: hepatitis, jaundice
hyperthermia
insomnia
mucous membrane irritation

muscle cramps
nausea
nitrophenols in blood and urine
psychosis
renal/urinary: nephritis, tubular
   necrosis, oliguria, pyuria, BUN
   elevated, albuminuria, biliuria,
   hematuria, urine casts and yellow
   stained urine, darkens rapidly on
   contact with air
respiratory: dyspnea, tachypnea,
   pulmonary edema, chest
   tightness, anoxia
sclera: yellow stained
sweating
tachycardia
thirst
vertigo
vomiting
weakness

Death due to hyperthermia,
   respiratory or circulatory failure

Chronic Exposure Effects

agranulocytosis
angina
anoxia
anxiety/sense of well-
   being
cataracts

conjunctivitis
cyanosis
dermal rash
headache
hepatic: hepatitis,
   jaundice

nitrophenols in blood
   or urine
peripheral neuritis
renal damage
sweating
thirst
weight loss

Suspected Effects

Dinocap:
  dermal: necrosis, sensitization 23
  reproductive system effects 22

Nitrofen:
  carcinogenesis 2(173), 11(279), 23,
    28
  mutagenesis 11(279), 23
  postnatal damage 23
  prenatal damage 11(277), 23
  reproductive system effects 23

Toxicology

Nitrophenols destroy cell membranes and uncouple oxidative phosphoryl-ation, resulting in increased oxidative metabolism and oxygen consumption and depletion of carbohydrate and fat stores. Metabolic activation and subsequent toxicity are increased by heat.

Active Ingredients

binapacryl	dinocap	DNOC
dinitroorthocresol	dinoseb	(dinitroorthocresol)
dinitrophenol	DNC	DNP (dinitrophenol)
dinobuton	(dinitroorthocresol)	nitrofen

Organochlorines ───────────────────────────

Class of Active Ingredients

> **Use:** acaricides, insecticides, molluscicides, nematicides, piscicides, and rodenticides

Acute Exposure Effects

abdominal pain
acidosis
agranulocytosis
ataxia
behavioral disturbances
bradycardia/tachycardia
cardiac arrhythmias
CNS stimulation followed by
   depression
coma
convulsions (epileptiform): may be
   delayed for weeks or months
cyanosis
delirium
dermal: dermatitis, facial
   congestion, purpura
diarrhea
dizziness
EEG disturbances
eye: irritation, visual disturbances
gastroenteritis
headache
hepatic injury

hypertension
hyperthermia
insomnia
leukocytosis
mucous membrane irritation
muscle twitching
nausea
pallor
paresis
paresthesia
renal/urinary: renal injury,
   albuminuria, anuria, hematuria
respiratory: cough, dyspnea,
   pulmonary edema, respiratory
   depression
salivation
sweating
thrombocytopenia
tremors
vomiting
weakness

Death due to respiratory failure

Chronic Exposure Effects

abdominal pain
anorexia/weight loss
chest pain
eye: nystagmus, visual disturbances
hepatic degeneration
hormonal disturbance
incoordination
insomnia
joint pain
mental changes

mutagenesis (toxaphene only 22)
myocardial irritability
paralysis
paresis
peripheral neuropathy
renal degeneration
splenomegaly
tremor
vertigo
weakness

Suspected Effects

Aldrin:
  carcinogenesis 5(384), 36
  reproductive system effects 2(150)

Chlordane:
  blood dyscrasias 12(58)
  carcinogenesis 12(57–58), 20
  mutagenesis 12(55)
  postnatal damage 12(54, 57)
  prenatal damage 12(57)
  reproductive system effects 12(54)

Chlordecone:
  carcinogenesis 22, 28
  prenatal damage 2(151), 4(A–19)
  reproductive system effects 2(151),
    4(A–19)

Chlorobenzilate:
  carcinogenesis 22

Dicofol:
  carcinogenesis 23

Dieldrin:
  carcinogenesis 5(384), 36
  reproductive system effects 2(150)

Endrin:
  mutagenesis 22
  prenatal damage 22

Heptachlor:
  carcinogenesis 23
  hyperreflexia 23

Lindane:
  anemia (aplastic) 12(222), 22, 36
  carcinogenesis 12(222), 22, 28
  postnatal damage 22
  prenatal damage 22

Methoxychlor:
  carcinogenesis 23
  growth reduction 23
  prenatal damage 2(150), 23
  reproductive system effects 2(150),
    23

Mirex:
  carcinogenesis 28
  reproductive system effects 23

Toxaphene:
  carcinogenesis 22, 28
  developmental effects 22
  reproductive system effects 22

Toxicology

Organochlorines interfere with axonal transmission of nerve impulses, thereby disrupting the function of the nervous system, primarily the central nervous system. They induce mixed function oxidases, protein and lipid synthesis, and changes in hepatic enzymes. Their toxicity varies considerably as a function of the degree of chlorination. They are stored in human and animal fat for long periods.

Methoxychlor mimics the effects of estradiol, which may affect fertility.

Additional Information

Most pesticides in this class are a mixture of structurally similar chemicals, e.g., toxaphene includes over 170 compounds that have 10 carbon atoms and 6 to 10 chlorine atoms. Its toxicity may vary with different formulations.

Photolysis of organochlorines may result in compounds that are more toxic than the original pesticide.

Active Ingredients

aldrin
benzene hexachloride
γ-benzene
   hexachloride
   (lindane)
BHC (benzene
   hexachloride)
γ-BHC (lindane)
camphechlor
   (toxaphene)
chlordane
chlordecone
chlorinated camphene
   (toxaphene)
chlorobenzilate
chlorophenothane
   (DDT)

chloropropylate
DDD (TDE)
DDT
dicofol
dicophane (DDT)
dieldrin
dienochlor
endosulfan
endrin
ethylan
HCH (benzene
   hexachloride)
γ-HCH (lindane)
heptachlor
hexachlorocylohexane
   (benzene
   hexachloride)

γ-hexachlorocyclo-
   hexane (lindane)
isobenzan
lindane
methoxychlor
methoxy-DDT
   (methoxychlor)
mirex
octachlorocamphene
   (toxaphene)
polychlorinated
   camphene
   (toxaphene)
TDE
tetrachlorodiphenylethane
   (TDE)
toxaphene

Organophosphates ──────────────────────

Class of Active Ingredients

Use: acaricides, fungicides, herbicides, insecticides, nematicides, rodenticides

Acute Exposure Effects

acidosis
alkyl phosphates in urine
anorexia
anoxia
aphasia
arreflexia
ataxia
cardiac: bradycardia/tachycardia,
    heart block
cholinesterase inhibition
CNS impairment
coma
confusion
convulsions
cyanosis
dermatitis
diarrhea
dizziness/vertigo
EEG and EMG disturbances
eye: miosis/mydriasis, loss of
    accomodation, ocular pain,
    sensation of retrobulbar pressure,
    tearing, dark or blurred vision,
    conjunctival hyperemia, cataracts
GI: abdominal cramps, heart burn,
    hyperperistalsis
hallucinations
headache
hepatic damage

hyperglycemia
hypertension/hypotension
hyperthermia
incontinence/tenesmus
leukopenia
muscle atrophy and twitching
nausea
pallor
paresis
paresthesias
psychosis
renal damage
respiratory: apnea, dyspnea,
    hypopnea, atelectasis,
    bronchoconstriction,
    bronchopharyngeal secretion,
    chest tightness, productive cough,
    rales/ronchi, wheezing,
    pulmonary edema, laryngeal
    spasms, rhinorrhea, oronasal
    frothing
salivation
shock
somnolence/insomnia
sweating
vomiting
weakness

Death due to respiratory failure

Chronic Exposure Effects
Same as Above Plus:
frontal lobe impairment

Suspected Effects
neurologic deficits
    7(290)

Suspected Effects (*continued*)

Azinphos Methyl:
  carcinogenesis 2(174), 22
Bensulide:
  hematocrit depressed 23
  hemoglobin depressed 23
  SAP, SGOT, SGPT elevated 23
  splenomegaly 23
Carbophenothion:
  prenatal damage 22
Chlorfenvinphos:
  mutagenesis 22
  prenatal damage 22
  reproductive system effects 22
Crufomate:
  paralysis 22
Cyanofenphos:
  neuropathy (delayed, peripheral)
    15(3)
DFP:
  neuropathy (delayed, peripheral)
    2(99)
Dichlorvos:
  carcinogenesis 23
  lung hemorrhage 23
  mutagenesis 2(201)
Dimethoate:
  carcinogenesis 22
  mutagenesis 22
  prenatal damage 22, 23
Disulfoton:
  prenatal damage 22
  splenic damage 23
EPBP:
  neuropathy (delayed, peripheral)
    15(3)
EPN:
  growth retardation 23
  neuropathy (delayed, peripheral)
    9(410), 15(3), 22
  prenatal damage 22
  splenomegaly 23
Leptophos:
  neuropathy (delayed, peripheral)
    9(411), 15(3)

Malathion:
  prenatal damage 23
Merphos®:
  paralysis 9(409)
Methidathion:
  prenatal damage 23
Mipafox:
  demyelination 7(291)
  paralysis 9(331)
Parathion:
  carcinogenesis 2(174), 23, 27
  prenatal damage 23
Phosmet:
  prenatal damage 22
Phosphamidon:
  mutagenesis 22
Pirimiphos-ethyl:
  prenatal damage 22
Pirimiphos-methyl:
  mutagenesis 22
Ronnel:
  carcinogenesis 20
  prenatal damage 20, 23
  reproductive system effects 22
Sulfotepp:
  Cheyne-Stokes respiration 20
Tetrachlorvinphos:
  carcinogenesis 22
  hemoglobin depression 22
  postnatal damage 22
Trichlorfon:
  carcinogenesis 22, 23, 36
  mutagenesis 2(200)
  neuropathy (delayed, peripheral) 22
  paralysis 9(355)
  prenatal damage 2(200), 22
  reproductive system effects 22
Trichloronat:
  may be contaminated with TCDD
    36 (see Chlorophenoxys for
    health effects of TCDD)

Toxicology

Acetylcholinesterase enzymes are inactivated by phosphorylation, causing an accumulation of acetylcholine at cholinergic neuro-effector and skeletal myoneural junctions and autonomic ganglia. The result is a combination of muscarinic and nicotinic effects. CNS function may also be impaired. Many organophosphates are readily converted from thions to more toxic oxons in the liver. Both oxons and thions are inactivated by hydrolysis. The hydrolysis products, alkyl phosphates and phenols, are readily excreted. Neurotoxic organophosphates cause axonal and myelin degeneration in distal fibers. Neural damage is possibly related to changes in tissue distribution of copper. Organophosphates are mild inducers of mixed function oxidases. Mutagenic and teratogenic properties may be the result of alkylation by organophosphates. Several members of this class are synergistic with each other. Commonly used hydrocarbon solvents may cause respiratory depression, thereby magnifying organophosphate toxicity.

Malathion toxicity is enhanced via by-products that are formed during storage.

Active Ingredients

acephate
Akton®
Aspon®
azinophosmethyl
bensophos
  (phosalone)
bensulide
Bomyl®
bromophos
carbophenthion
chlorfenvinphos
chlormephos
chlorphoxim
chlorpyrifos
chlorthiophos
coumaphos
crotoxyphos
crufomate
cyanofenphos
cyanophos
DDVP (dichlorvos)
DEF®
demeton
demeton methyl

demeton-*O*-methyl
  sulfoxide
  (oxydemeton-
  methyl)
DFP
dialifor (dialifos)
dialifos
Diazinon®
dicapthon
dichlorvos
dichlofenthion
dicrotophos
diisopropyl
  fluorophosphate
  (DFP)
dimefox
dimephenthoate
  (phenthoate)
dimethoate
dioxathion
disulfoton
edifenphos
endothion
EPBP

EPN
ethion
ethoprop
ethyl parathion
  (parathion)
famphur
fenamiphos
fenitrothion
fensulfothion
fenthion
fonophos
formothion
fosthietan
IBP
iodofenfos (jodfenfos)
isofenphos
isofluorphage (DFP)
isoxathion
jodfenfos
leptophos
malathion
mephosfolan
Merphos®
methamidophos

Active Ingredients (*continued*)

methidathion
methyl demeton
  (demeton-methyl)
methyl parathion
methyl systox
Methyl Trithion®
mevinphos
mipafox
monocrotophos
naled
nephocarp
  (carbophenothion)
oxydemeton methyl
parathion
parathion methyl
phencapton
phenthoate
phorate

phorazetim
phosalone
phosfolan
phosmet
phosphamide
  (dimethoate)
phosphamidon
phoxim
pirimiphos-ethyl
pirimiphos-methyl
profenfos
propaphos
propetamphos
prothoate
pyrazophos
pyridaphenthion
pyrophosphate

quinalphos
ronnel
schradan
stirofos
sulfotepp
sulprofos
temephos
TEPP
terbufos
tetrachlorvinphos
tetraethylpyrophosphate
  (TEPP)
thiometon
timet (phorate)
triazophos
trichlorfon
trichloronate

Organosulfurs

Class of Active Ingredients

Use: acaricides, fungicides, herbicides, insecticides, miticides

Acute Exposure Effects

coma
conjunctivitis
dermal irritation
dizziness
drowsiness

headache
hematuria
nausea
proteinuria
pulmonary edema

respiratory depression
sensory loss
unconsciousness
vomiting

Chronic Exposure Effects

anorexia/weight loss
conjunctivitis
cough

hypotension
incoordination
nausea

Suspected Effects

Aramite®:
carcinogenesis 28, 36
Chlorfenson:
hepatic effects 9(623)
splenic hemorrhage 9(623)
thyroid effects 9(623)

Propargite:
carcinogenesis 22
hepatomegaly 22
lymph node abnormalities 22
prenatal damage 22
renal weight increase 22

Toxicology

Organosulfurs:

—interfere with electron transport;
—block an enzyme in the respiratory pathway between acetate and citrate;
—may function as a general receptor for hydrogen in redox reactions, producing hydrogen sulfide.

Active Ingredients

Aramite®
chlorfenson
difenson (chlorfenson)

fenson
ovex (chlorfenson)
propargite

tetradifon
tetrasul

Organotins ———————————————————————

Class of Active Ingredients

Use: acaricides, fungicides, insecticides, mulluscicides

Acute Exposure Effects

abdominal pain
anuria
cerebral edema
CNS damage
dermal: irritation, burns, dermatitis
diarrhea
dizziness
eye: irritation, conjunctival edema,
    tearing, photophobia
GI disturbance
headache
hyperthermia
nausea
paralysis
respiratory: irritation, cough,
    pharyngitis, pulmonary edema,
    rhinorrhea
vomiting
weakness

Chronic Exposure Effects
Chronic effects may exist, but no data were found.

Suspected Effects
Cyhexatin:
    carcinogenesis 36
    reproductive effects 22
Fenbutatin Oxide:
    anorexia 23
    postnatal damage 22
    prenatal damage 22, 23
    weight depression 23

Fentin Acetate, Chloride, and Hydroxide:
    cerebral edema 36
    leukocytopenia 22, 36
    reproductive system effects 22, 36

Toxicology
Organotins inhibit oxidative phosphorylation and α-keto oxidases.

Active Ingredients
cyhexatin
fenbutatin oxide
fentin acetate
fentin chloride
fentin hydroxide
triphenyltin acetate
    (fentin acetate)
triphenyltin hydroxide
    (fentin hydroxide)

Oxyfluorfen _____

Active Ingredient

> **Use:** herbicide

Suspected Effects

carcinogenesis 22	mutagenesis 22	renal tubular
enzyme changes 22	pigmented liver cells	vacuolization 22
hepatomegaly 22	in bile 22	

Hepatocellular carcinoma may be due to the impurity perchloroethylene 22 (see Perchloroethylene under Halocarbon Fumigants)

Pentachloronitrobenzene ————————————————————

Active Ingredient

> **Synonym:** PCNB
> **Use:** fungicide

Acute Exposure Effects
  eye: conjunctivitis, corneal damage

Chronic Exposure Effects
Effects may occur, but no data were found.

Suspected Effects
  bone marrow changes 36   methemoglobinemia 9(586)
  carcinogenesis 9(587), 22, 26, 27, 36   mutagenesis 9(587), 27
  dermal irritation 9(587)   prenatal damage 9(587), 22, 26, 27,
  hepatic abnormalities 36   36

Toxicology
PCNB is metabolized to pentachloroaniline and methylpentachlorophenol sul-
fite. The latter may be responsible for prenatal damage. Hexachlorobenzene, a
frequent contaminant of pentachloronitrobenzene, may also be responsible for
prenatal damage and carcinogenesis (see Hexachlorobenzene).

Pentachlorophenol ────────────────────

Active Ingredient

Synonym: PCP
Use: fungicide, herbicide, insecticide, molluscicide

Acute Exposure Effects

abdominal pain
acidosis
anorexia
cardiac dilation
CNS injury
coma
convulsions
cyanosis
dehydration
dermal: chloracne, flushing,
   irritation, dermatitis
dizziness
edema (cerebral)
eye: irritation, scotoma
GI upset
headache
heat sensitivity
hepatic: hepatomegaly,
   degeneration
hyperthermia
irritability followed by lethargy

leukocytosis
mental deterioration
metabolic rate elevation
mucous membrane irritation
muscle weakness and spasm
nausea
renal/urinary: albuminuria,
   glycosuria, azotemia, tubular
   degeneration, polyuria/oliguria
respiratory: tachypnea, chest pain,
   coughing, dyspnea, congestion,
   sneezing
stupor
sweating
tachycardia
thirst
vomiting

Death due to cardiac failure,
   respiratory failure, or hyperthermia

Chronic Exposure Effects

anemia
dermal: chloracne,
   dermatitis
hepatic damage

leukopenia
metabolic rate
   elevation
peripheral neuropathy
   (neuritis, neuralgia)

pulmonary damage
renal damage
weight loss

Suspected Effects

carcinogenesis 27
hyperglycemia 3(2606)
hyperperistalsis 3(2606)
hypertension 3(2606)
mutagenesis 9(475)

porphyria 9(475)
postnatal damage 3(2608), 9(475),
   27
prenatal damage 3(2608), 9(475),
   22, 27

Toxicology

Pentachlorophenol:

—causes gross damage to mitochondria;
—inactivates respiratory enzymes;
—uncouples oxidative phosphorylation;
—inhibits myosin ATP;
—induces hepatic enzymes.

Inadequate opportunity for heat loss and increase in body temperature may lead to fatal hyperthermia. Children often manifest dehydration and acidosis following exposure.

Additional Information

The effects of pentachlorophenol mimic those of nitrophenols and organophosphates. High external temperature is synergistic with PCP.

PCP is frequently contaminated with the extremely toxic polychlorinated dibenzodioxins and dibenzofurans (see the Chlorophenoxy class for a discussion of dioxins).

Petroleum Distillates _____

Class of Active and Inert Ingredients

Use: inert ingredients, insecticides

Petroleum distillates include numerous compounds with wide-ranging chemical structures and properties. The designation "petroleum distillates" on a label is insufficient to predict most health effects. For example, it may include the relatively innocuous paraffins or the highly toxic benzene compounds. If a poisoning has occurred, it is necessary to obtain information from the manufacturer on the specific type of distillates used in order to assess their health impact.

Detailed information can be obtained elsewhere in this book on the following: benzene, cyclohexane, cyclohexanone, halocarbons, kerosene, methyl ketones, mineral spirits, petroleum ether, rubber solvent, stoddard solvent, toluene, varnish makers' and painters' naphtha, and xylene.

Acute Exposure Effects

albuminuria
anorexia
cardiac arrhythmias
CNS depression
constipation
cyanosis
dermal: irritation,
  itching, burning,
  rash
eye discomfort

headache
hematuria
hepatic damage
hyperreflexia
hypothermia
insomnia
mucous membrane
  irritation
narcosis

nausea
nervousness
paresthesia
psychic disturbances
respiratory: choking,
  coughing,
  pneumonitis
tachycardia
vomiting

Chronic Exposure Effects

anorexia
cardiac disturbances
dermal: drying,
  cracking, rash,
  pruritus, dermatitis,
  itching
diarrhea/constipation
drowsiness

eye discomfort
GI upset, cramps
headache (chronic)
hyperreflexia
insomnia
nausea
nervousness
numbness

paresthesia
syncopal attacks
tachypnea
throat: burning
  sensations, dryness
vertigo
weakness

Suspected Effects

fainting 24(34)
weight loss 24(34)

Toxicology
Petroleum distillates are fat solvents that cause cellular and tissue damage including demyelination and axonal degeneration of peripheral nerves, destruction of cell membranes, fatty degeneration of muscle fibers, neurogenic atrophy, and the rupture of Schwann cell membranes. CNS depression is a rapid manifestation. Dermal exposure causes histamine release from nerve endings leading to the accumulation of metabolic products and irritation of exposed areas.

Increased chain length generally leads to symptoms which are more severe and persistent. The higher the carbon number, the greater the anesthetic activity of its vapor and the likelihood of respiratory irritation and arrest. One and two carbon chains are simple asphyxiants which do not usually cause general systemic effects.

If hydrocarbons are aspirated during induced emesis, a small amount can coat the lungs and cause rapid severe pneumonitis, pulmonary edema, and hemorrhage.

Active and Inert Ingredients
Note: All of the following are both active and inert ingredients:

aliphatic petroleum derivatives	petroleum distillates
aromatic petroleum derivatives	xylene range aromatic solvent
paraffins	

Petroleum Ether

Inert Ingredient

Synonym: ligroin

Acute Exposure Effects

anemia
cerebral edema
clonic convulsions
CNS depression
cold sensations in
  extremities
coma
dermatitis
dizziness
drowsiness
eye irritation

fatigue
headache
hematuria
mucous membrane
  irritation
paresthesias
proteinuria
respiratory: coughing,
  irritation, dyspnea,
  bronchial
  pneumonia,
  depression, failure

vision blurred
vomiting
unconsciousness
weakness

Death due to respiratory
  failure

Chronic Exposure Effects

anemia
anorexia
dizziness
hematuria
nervousness

neuromuscular: demyelination of
  nerves and axonal degeneration,
  polyneuropathy, paresthesia, pain
  in limbs
photosensitivity
proteinuria
weakness
weight loss

Toxicology

Petroleum ether is a fat solvent that casuses CNS dysfunction and the destruction of other tissues.

Phenol ───────────────────────────

Inert Ingredient

Synonyms: carbolic acid, hydroxybenzene

Acute Exposure Effects

CNS disturbances
collapse
coma
convulsions
dermal: anesthesia, whitening,
   corrosion, gangrene
dyspnea
eye: irritation, conjunctival
   swelling, corneal whitening,
   hypesthesia, blindness
frothing from nose and mouth
headache
hepatic damage
hypertension followed by
   hypotension
hypothermia
mucous membrane irritation
muscle weakness and tremors
myocardial depression
pallor
renal damage
salivation
shock
tachycardia followed by
   bradycardia
tinnitus
urine: darkened, phenol levels
   elevated, phenyl sulfate and
   phenyl glucuronide present
vasoconstriction (peripheral)

Chronic Exposure Effects

anorexia
dermal: rash,
   ochronosis
diarrhea
dizziness
dysphagia
fainting
GI disturbances
hepatic: tenderness,
   damage,
   hepatomegaly
mental disturbances
muscle pain
nervous disorders
renal damage
urine darkened
vertigo
vomiting
weakness
weight loss

Suspected Effects

blood: cells vacuolized, hyalinized,
   or hypergranulated 3(2570)
carcinogenesis 27
genitourinary damage 3(2570)
muscle fiber striation 3(2570)
papillomas 25
paralysis 25
parenchymatous nephritis 3(2570)
prenatal damage 27
respiratory: hyperemia, infarcts,
   pneumonia, hyperplasia of the
   peribronchial tissues, purulent
   bronchitis 3(2570)

Toxicology

Phenol is a fat solvent that causes CNS dysfunction and the destruction of
other tissues. It is oxidized and conjugated with sulfuric, glucuronic, and other
acids and excreted in urine as free or conjugated phenol.

Additional Information

Individuals with convulsive disorders, or skin, respiratory, liver, or kidney
problems are at higher risk when exposed to phenol.

o-Phenylphenol _____

Active Ingredient

Use: fungicide

Suspected Effects
carcinogenesis 11(339)

dermal irritation
(severe) 26

eye irritation (severe)
26

mutagenesis 27

prenatal damage 27

Other effects may occur, but no data were found.

Phosphine and Phosphides ————————————————

Class of Active Ingredients

Use: fumigants, rodenticides

Exposure Effects

abdominal pain
acidosis
anorexia
ataxia
bilirubinemia
breath: garlic odor
cerebral edema
CNS depression
coma
convulsions
cyanosis
dermal injury
diarrhea
dizziness
drowsiness
dysphagia
EKG abnormalities
eye: double vision, pain, tearing
fatigue
hallucinations
headache
hemorrhage
hepatic damage: elevated serum
    GOT, GPT, LDH, and alkaline
    phosphatase, jaundice, fatty
    degeneration, necrosis, and
    hepatomegaly
hypercalcemic tetany
hyperthermia
hypotension

meteorism
methemoglobinemia
mucous membrane irritation
myocarditis
nausea
pallor
palpitations
prothrombinemia
renal/urinary: tubular necrosis,
    albuminuria, uremia, anuria,
    hematuria
respiratory: bronchospasm, chest
    tightness, coughing of frothy
    fluid, dyspnea, depression,
    hyperemia, rales, laryngeal and
    pulmonary edema
rhinorrhagia
tachycardia
tenesmus
thirst
throat dryness
thrombocytopenia
tremor
vertigo
vomiting
weakness

Death due to pulmonary edema,
    cardiac arrest, circulatory collapse,
    or respiratory failure

Toxicology

Phosphides react with water and hydrochloride in the stomach to produce phosphine gas (PH_3).

Active Ingredients

aluminum phosphide
hydrogen phosphide
    (phosphine)
magnesium phosphide

phosphide
phosphine
zinc phosphide

Picloram ———————————————————

Active Ingredient

> **Synonym:** agent white
> **Use:** herbicide

Exposure Effects
dermal irritation
eye irritation
nausea

nervous system
  disorders
respiratory tract
  irritation

Suspected Effects
carcinogenesis 2(174),
  20, 27
hepatic damage 23
leukopenia 27

prenatal damage 27
reproductive system
  damage 23

Toxicology
Picloram uncouples oxidative phosphorylation.

Piperonyl Butoxide ————————————————

Active Ingredient

Use: pesticide synergist

Suspected Effects

anorexia 9(114)

carcinogenesis 27, 36

coma 9(114)

convulsions 9(115)

dermal irritation
  9(114)

hepatic damage 9(116)

hyperexcitability
  9(115)

prenatal damage 27

prostration 9(114)

renal damage 9(116)

tearing 9(114)

unsteadiness 9(114)

vomiting 9(114)

weight loss 9(115)

Toxicology

Piperonyl butoxide inhibits microsomal enzymes. It potentiates diethyl substituted phosphorothionates (parathion and azinphosethyl) and antagonizes dimethyl substituted compounds.

Additional Information

Piperonyl butoxide is commonly used with pyrethrins and rotenone.

Pronamide ——————————————————————

Active Ingredient

Use: herbicide

Exposure Effects
eye and mucous membrane
irritation

Suspected Effects
carcinogenesis
21(637), 22, 23, 27

Other effects may occur, but no data were found.

Toxicology
Pronamide inhibits mitosis.

Propylene Oxide _____

Active and Inert Ingredient

Synonym: methyloxirane
Use: fumigant

Acute Exposure Effects

abdominal pain
anesthesia
ataxia
CNS depression
convulsions
cyanosis
dermal: dermatitis, burns
diarrhea
dizziness
eye: burns, irritation, conjunctivitis,
    tearing, double vision, injury
headache
hepatic damage
mucous membrane irritation
nausea

renal damage
respiratory: irritation, hoarseness,
    substernal pressure, chest pain,
    laryngeal and pulmonary edema,
    bronchospasm, respiratory
    depression, dyspnea, pneumonia,
    coughing of frothy fluid
tremor
unconsciousness
vomiting
weakness

Death due to pulmonary edema or
    respiratory failure

Chronic Exposure Effects

infection due to increased
    susceptibility
respiratory irritation

Suspected Effects

carcinogenesis 20, 27
mutagenesis 27

Additional Information

Solutions more dilute than 10% may produce greater dermal toxicity than
more concentrated solutions.

Persons with respiratory disorders may be at greater risk following exposure.

Pyrazon ⎯⎯⎯⎯⎯⎯⎯⎯⎯⎯⎯⎯⎯⎯⎯⎯⎯⎯⎯

Active Ingredient

> **Synonym:** chloridazon
> **Use:** herbicide

Suspected Effects

ataxia 9(567)	hypothermia 9(567)	pulmonary disorders
convulsions 9(567)	excitability 9(567)	9(567)
hypotension 9(567)	prenatal damage 27	tremors 27

Other effects may occur, but no data were found.

Pyrethrins and Pyrethroids ━━━━━━━━━━━━━

Class of Active Ingredients

Use: insecticides

Acute Exposure Effects

ataxia
convulsions leading to muscle
   fibrillation and paralysis
dermal: dermatitis, edema
diarrhea
dyspnea
headache
hepatic microsomal enzyme
   induction
irritability
peripheral vascular collapse

pyrethrins or pyrethroids in urine
   or feces
rhinorrhea
serum alkaline phosphatase levels
   elevated
tinnitus
tremors
vomiting

Death due to respiratory failure

Allergic reactions have included the following effects:

anaphylaxis
bronchospasm
eosinophilia
fever
hypersensitivity pneumonia (cough,
   dyspnea, fever, lung infiltrates)
pallor

pollinosis
sweating
swelling (sudden): face, eyelids, lips,
   mucous membranes (oral and
   laryngeal)
tachycardia

Chronic Exposure Effects
Chronic effects may exist, but no data were found.

Suspected Effects
cyclic GMP increase in brain
   (especially the cerebellum) 9(81)
hepatomegaly 15(43)
Bioresmethrin:
   hepatic damage 36
   prenatal damage 36
Decamethrin:
   choreoathetosis 9(80)
   hypotension 9(80)
   prenatal damage 9(81)
   shock 9(80)
Dimethrin:
   anorexia/weight loss 36
   stupor 36

hyperplasia of bile duct 15(43)
tearing (bloody) 15(43)
urinary incontinence 15(43)
Fenvalerate:
   albuminemia 23
   carcinogenesis 23
   eye: conjunctivitis, corneal opacity
   23
   lymph node damage 23
   splenic damage 23
   Wallerian nerve damage 23
   weight loss 23

Suspected Effects (*continued*)

Permethrin:
carcinogenesis 22
food consumption reduced 22
hepatomegaly 22
neural demyelination 22
prenatal damage 22

Tetramethrin:
carcinogenesis 23

Toxicology

Pyrethrins and pyrethroids block nerve impulse transmissions by repetitive firing of nerve motor end plates through repeated presynaptic nerve terminal depolarizations. They inhibit sodium/potassium conduction in the nerve cells and induce liver microsomal enzymes.

Additional Information

Persons with a history of allergy or asthma are particularly reactive to pyrethrins. Children are more sensitive than adults.

Active Ingredients

allethrin	fenopropathrin	phenothrin
barthrin	fenvalerate	pyrethrin
bioresmethrin	flucythrinate	resmethrin
cypermethrin	fluvalinate	tetramethrin
decamethrin	jasmolin	*d*-transallethrin
dimethrin	permethrin	

Pyridine

Inert Ingredient

Acute Exposure Effects

back pain
CNS: disturbances,
    depression,
dermal: irritation,
    photosensitization
diarrhea
dizziness
eye irritation

GI upset
headache
hepatic damage
insomnia
mucous membrane
    irritation
narcosis
nausea

nervousness
pyridine and N-
    methyl-pyridinium
    hydroxide in urine
renal damage
urinary frequency
weakness

Chronic Exposure Effects

anorexia
back pain (lower)
CNS disturbances
    (transient)
diarrhea
dizziness

GI disturbances
headache
hepatic damage
insomnia
mental dullness
nausea

nervousness
renal damage
urinary frequency
vertigo
vomiting

Suspected Effects

CNS aphasia, diffused cortical
    affliction 3(2730)
corneal damage 3(2729)

mutagenesis 27
paralysis 27
prenatal damage 3(2729)

Toxicology

Pyridine is a fat solvent that causes CNS disturbances and the destruction of other tissues. It releases cyanide when heated (see Cyanides).

Red Squill

Active Ingredient

Use: rodenticide

Acute Exposure Effects

abdominal pain
anorexia
blood: eosinophilia; elevated
  glycosides, potassium, and
  calcium levels
cardiac: hemorrhage, bradycardia,
  palpitations, heart block
CNS depression
convulsions
delirium
dermal rash (uticarial or
  scarlatiniform)
diarrhea
disorientation

eye: amblyopia, photophobia, loss
  of visual acuity, flashing, halos,
  scotoma, color vision aberrations
neuralgia
hallucinations
headache
hypotension
mental disorders
nausea
nightmares
vertigo
vomiting
weakness

Death due to cardiac arrest or
  ventricular fibrillation

Chronic Exposure Effects

blood: depression of potassium,
  calcium, and platelet levels
breast development in men
EKG abnormalities
gastrointestinal disorders

paralysis
renal injury
visual disturbances
weakness

Toxicology

Red squill, a cardiac glycoside, mimics the toxic syndrome of digitalis poisoning. It inhibits Na^+ and K^+-activated ATPase in cell membranes, which impairs the active cation transport mechanism. This results in a gradual intracellular potassium loss and sodium gain. Infants and children may be less susceptible to red squill than adults. Toxic effects are more severe in persons with hypothyroidism, kidney disease, heart disease, any circumstance causing decreased potassium levels (diuretic users), increased calcium levels, and those using ephedrine. Cardiac effects may persist for 2–3 weeks following acute exposures.

Visual disturbances may be due to transient retrobulbar optic neuritis or visual cortex damage.

Additional Information

Red squill contains a number of cardiac glycosides: scillaren A, scillaren B, and scilliroside.

Rotenone ——————————————————————————

Active Ingredient

Synonyms: cube, derris, nicouline, tubatoxin
Use: acaricide, insecticide, piscicide

Acute Exposure Effects
abdominal pain
anosmia
bradycardia
coma
convulsions
dermal: dermatitis,
   sensitivity reactions
dysphasia

eye irritation
GI irritation
metallic taste
mucous membrane
   inflammation and
   numbness
nausea

respiratory
   stimulation
   followed by
   depression
stupor
tremor
vomiting

Chronic Exposure Effects
hepatic damage
limb paralysis
rash
renal damage

Suspected Effects
carcinogenesis 9(85), 27
congestive heart failure 9(85)
hypoglycemia 9(84)
incoordination 9(85)
mutagenesis 20, 27
mydriasis 9(85)

postnatal damage 9(84)
prenatal damage 9(84), 20
pulmonary congestion 9(85)
pulse: feeble 9(85)
soft palate destruction 9(85)
ulcerative keratitis 9(85)

Toxicology
Rotenoids inhibit the oxidation of NAD, thus blocking oxidative phosphorylation. They also block nerve conduction.

Additional Information
Rotenone is one of six naturally occurring rotenoids that can be extracted from derris root and cube. Information regarding the mammalian toxicity of the other five rotenoids is not complete. However, they are insecticidal and will appear in rotenone preparations.

Rubber Solvent ―――――――――――――――――――――

Inert Ingredient

> **Composition:** 0.1% monolefin, 1.5% benzene, 3.4% alkyl benzene, 41.4% paraffins, 53.6% monocycloparaffins

Acute Exposure Effects

anemia	headache	respiratory: coughing,
ataxia	hematopoietic:	irritation, bronchial
CNS depression	leukemia, aplastic	pneumonia,
coma	anemia, leukopenia	depression
convulsions	hematuria	vomiting
dermatitis	mucous membrane	weakness
dizziness	irritation	weight loss
drowsiness	nausea	
eye irritation	proteinuria	Death due to respiratory
fatigue		failure

Delayed-onset anorexia has occurred months after acute exposures.

Chronic Exposure Effects

anemia	hematuria	proteinuria
dermal: chapping and	nervousness	weakness
photosensitivity	pain in limbs	weight loss
dizziness	peripheral neuropathy	

Suspected Effects

conjunctivitis 27	hepatic hyperplasia	respiratory:
motor activity changes	24(84)	pulmonary
27		hemorrhage and
		perivascular edema
		24(85)

Toxicology

Rubber solvent is a fat solvent that causes CNS dysfunction and the destruction of other tissues. Peripheral neuropathy following chronic exposures has been attributed to the hexane fraction of rubber solvent. Hematopoietic diseases may result from the benzene fraction.

Additional Information

For additional information on the benzene constituent of rubber solvent, see Benzene.

Sodium Chlorate

Active Ingredient

Use: rodenticide

Acute Exposure Effects

abdominal pain
apathy
cardiac arrhythmias
chest pain
CNS depression
collapse
convulsions
cyanosis
dermal irritation
eye irritation

GI irritation
hemoglobinemia
hemolysis
hepatomegaly
hypotension
lumbar pain
methemoglobinemia
nausea
oral-pharyngeal
   membrane swelling

renal/urinary:
   azotemia, nephritis,
   tubular injury,
   albuminuria,
   anuria, darkened
   urine, hematuria
splenomegaly
vomiting

Death from
   hyperkalemia, renal
   failure, or
   methemoglobinemia

Chronic Exposure Effects
Chronic effects may exist, but no data were found.

Suspected Effects
mutagenesis 27

Sodium Fluoroacetate _____

Active Ingredient

Use: rodenticide

Acute Exposure Effects

anxiety
cardiac irregularities: irregular
    pulse, ectopic heartbeat,
    tachycardia, ventricular
    fibrillation
citrate accumulation in tissues
CNS disturbances
coma
convulsions
cyanosis
epigastric distress
excitation/depression
eye: blurred vision, nystagmus,
    miosis/mydriasis
hallucination (auditory)
hemorrhage (petechial)
hypotension

hypothermia
incontinence (fecal)
nausea
organ congestion
paresis
paresthesia
renal tubular degeneration
respiratory: depression, pulmonary
    edema, respiration irregular
salivation
spinal pressure
twitching of face
vomiting

Death due to respiratory depression
    or ventricular fibrillation

Chronic Exposure Effects
Chronic effects may exist, but no data were found.

Toxicology
The metabolite fluorocitrate blocks the tricarboxylic acid cycle by inhibiting
aconitase. This leads to the accumulation of citrate. Oxidative energy metabolism is inhibited, and CNS and cardiac functions are disturbed.

Additional Information
There is a latent period before effects appear.

Stoddard Solvent ─────────────────────────

Inert Ingredient

> **Composition:** 0.1% benzene, 0.5% indans and tetralins, 11.6% dicyclo paraffins, 14.1% alkyl benzene, 26% mono-cyclo paraffins, 47.7% paraffins

Acute Exposure Effects

CNS depression
coma
convulsions
dermal: rash, purple discoloration,
   dermatitis, pallor
dizziness
eye irritation
fatigue
fever
headache
hepatic: damage, jaundice

mucous membrane irritation
nausea
olfactory fatigue
pallor
respiratory: coughing, pneumonia
   bloody sputum, pulmonary
   edema, depression
uterine bleeding
vomiting
weakness

Chronic Exposure Effects

anemia (hemolytic
   and aplastic)
BUN elevated
cerebral hemmorhage
dermal: dermatitis,
   purple discoloration
dizziness
eye irritation

fatigue
headache
hepatic: damage,
   jaundice
hypoplasia of bone
   marrow
leukopenia

mucous membrane
   irritation
nervousness
pain in limbs
paresthesias
thrombocytopenia
weakness
weight loss

Suspected Effects

renal damage 3(3378)
uterine bleeding
   24(138)

Toxicology

The toxicology of Stoddard solvent is complex due to the numerous chemicals it contains (see Benzene and Petroleum distillates). The relative amounts of these chemicals determine the response characteristics. Stoddard solvent is a fat solvent that causes CNS dysfunction and the destruction of other tissues.

Strychnine ─────────────────────────────

Active Ingredient

Use: rodenticide

Acute Exposure Effects

anoxia
apprehension
CNS damage
convulsions
cyanosis
eye: miosis/mydriasis
exhaustion
facial grimace
hyperexcitability
hyperreflexia
opisthotonus
paralysis
perception: heightened acuity

restlessness
stiffness of face and neck muscles
strychnine in liver, kidney, and
    urine
sweating
thirst
violent motor reactions to sensory
    stimuli
vomiting (rare)

Death due to asphyxia and respiratory
    failure

Chronic Exposure Effects
Chronic effects may occur, but no data were found.

Suspected Effects
cholinesterase
    inhibition 9(98)
postnatal damage 27
prenatal damage 27

Toxicology
Strychnine blocks the inhibitory effects of Renshaw cells on motor cells to the spinal cord. This lowers the threshold for stimulation of the spinal nerves, causing hyperreflexia. Strychnine may inhibit cholinesterase.

Sulfur Dioxide ─────────────────

Active Ingredient

Use: fumigant

Acute Exposure Effects
anesthesia
CNS depression
convulsions
cyanosis
dermatitis
dizziness
eye: conjunctivitis, tearing, corneal
  burns, corneal opacity, double
  vision
headache
mucous membrane irritation
nausea

respiratory: depression, wheezing,
  hoarseness, substernal pain,
  dyspnea, bronchopneumonia,
  bronchoconstriction, rales,
  increased pulmonary resistance,
  laryngeal and pulmonary edema,
  bronchospasm, changes in
  pulmonary vascular resistance,
  coughing of frothy fluid
tremor
unconsciousness
weakness

Death due to pulmonary edema or
  respiratory failure

Chronic Exposure Effects
dermal: sensitization, burns
eye: corneal opacification and burns
erythropoietic stimulation
fatigue

respiratory: nasopharyngitis, throat
  dryness, cough, bronchitis,
  dyspnea, rhinorrhea, rhinitis
  rhinorrhagia
sense of smell altered

Suspected Effects
carcinogenesis 20, 26,
  27
mutagenesis 27
postnatal damage 27

prenatal damage 27
reproductive system
  damage 27

Additional Information
Ten to twenty percent of adults are hypersusceptible. Others often adapt and
exhibit few symptoms during chronic exposure.

Sulfuryl Fluoride ─────────────────────────────

Active Ingredient

Use: fumigant, insecticide

Acute Exposure Effects

abdominal pain
CNS depression
convulsions
dermal itching
dizziness
drowsiness
eye: conjunctivitis, double vision
headache
hepatic damage
mucous membrane irritation
muscle twitching
nausea

paresthesia
renal/urinary: renal injury,
    azotemia, proteinuria
respiratory: pharyngitis, laryngeal
    edema, bronchospasm,
    respiratory depression, rhinitis
vomiting
tremor
weakness

Death due to respiratory failure

Chronic Exposure Effects
Chronic effects may occur, but no data were found

Thiabendazole ───────────────

Active Ingredient

Use: fungicide, helminthicide

Acute Exposure Effects

angioedema	dizziness	lethargy
anorexia	epigastric distress	liver function changes
body odor	fainting	nausea
chills	fever	numbness
dermal: flushing,	headache	tinnitus
itching, rash	hyperglycemia	vomiting
diarrhea	hypotension	xanthopsia

Chronic Exposure Effects

Chronic effects may occur, but no data were found.

Suspected Effects

anemia 9(613)
bone marrow
   suppression 9(613)

mutagenesis 27
prenatal damage 27

Thiadiazins

Class of Active Ingredients

Use: fungicides, herbicides

Acute Exposure Effects

dermal irritation
diarrhea
dyspnea
eye irritation

respiratory tract
  irritation
tremors
vomiting
weakness

Suspected Effects
Ethazol:
body weight depression 22

Active Ingredients
bentazon
ethazol (etridiazol)
etridiazol

Thiocarbamates ————————————————————

Class of Active Ingredients

Use: fungicides, herbicides

The thiocarbamates have been divided into two subclasses, designated A and B.

A. Dithiocarbamates

Exposure Effects
See Carbon Disulfide for additional effects.

anorexia/weight loss
ataxia
CNS damage
coma
confusion
dermal: irritation, dermatitis,
    sensitization, uticaria
diarrhea
dizziness
drowsiness
eye: irritation, conjunctivitis
headache
hyporeflexia

hypothermia
lethargy
mucous membrane irritation
muscle weakness
nausea
paralysis
respiratory: cough, hoarseness,
    pneumonitis, nasal stuffiness,
    rhinitis, sneezing
vomiting

Death due to respiratory
    paralysis

Thiram, ferbam, metham, nabam, and ziram may be synergistic with alcohol producing the following effects (in addition to the above):

aldehyde
    dehydrogenase
    inhibition
cardiac arrhythmias
circulatory failure
convulsions

flushing
hypotension
myocardial ischemia
palpitation
peripheral
    vasodilation

respiratory:
    depression, dyspnea,
    chest tightness
shock
sweating
tachycardia
warm sensations

Suspected Effects
Ferbam:
carcinogenesis 27, 36
peripheral neuropathy (reversible)
    2(96–7)
postnatal damage 27
prenatal damage 27

Maneb:
antithyroid effects 9(601)
carcinogenesis 9(608), 10(145), 22,
    36
GI disturbances 9(607)
mutagenesis 22

Suspected Effects (*continued*)
Maneb (*continued*)
  prenatal damage 5(394), 9(608)
  renal damage 9(607)
  reproductive system effects 2(156),
    9(608)
  tremors 9(607)
  weakness 9(607)
Nabam:
  carcinogenesis 5(394), 36(70,76)
  goiter 5(394), 36(70,76)
  mutagenesis 5(394), 27, 36(70,76)
  prenatal damage 5(394), 27,
    36(70,76)
  reproductive system effects 27
Thiram:
  anemia 36
  blood coagulation depression 9(604)
  carcinogenesis 27, 36
  CNS demyelination 8(311), 15(38)
  GI hyperemia 8(311)
  GI irritation 15(38)
  GI ulceration 8(311)
  hematopoiesis suppression 9(604)
  hepatic necrosis 8(311), 15(38)
  immunosuppression 9(604)
  leukopenia 9(604)
  peripheral neuropathy (reversible)
    2(96), 8(311), 15(38)
  postnatal damage 9(604), 27

Thiram (*continued*)
  prenatal damage 9(604), 27, 36
  psychosis 15(38)
  renal necrosis 8(311), 15(38)
  reproductive system effects 9(604),
    27
  splenic necrosis 15(38)
  thrombocytopenia 9(604)
  thyroid damage 36
Zineb:
  alopecia 9(609)
  antithyroid effects 9(601)
  carcinogenesis 10(253), 22, 36
  hyperactivity/inactivity 9(609)
  muscle tone loss 9(609)
  mutagenesis 22, 27
  prenatal damage 5(394), 9(610),
    10(251), 22, 36
  reproductive system effects 2(156),
    27
Ziram:
  carcinogenesis 27, 36
  convulsions 9(606)
  peripheral neuropathy (reversible)
    2(96)
  prenatal damage 9(607), 36
  reproductive system effects 9(607)

Toxicology
Dithiocarbamates are partially metabolized to carbon disulfide, which is a neurotoxin (see Carbon Disulfide). They are not cholinesterase inhibitors.

Nabam, maneb, and zineb are metabolized to ethylene thiourea, which can cause carcinogenesis (liver, thyroid), goiter, mutagenesis, and teratogenesis 2(187,189), 5(394), 22, 36(70,76).

Ferbam, thiram, and ziram may be metabolized to nitrosamines, which are carcinogenic 36.

B. Monothiocarbamates

Exposure Effects
  cough
  dermal irritation
  eye irritation
  respiratory mucous membrane
    irritation
  sneezing

Suspected Effects
  paralysis 15(38)

Cycloate:
  dermal edema 9(539)
  dermal hyperemia 9(539)
Diallate:
  carcinogenesis 10(73), 22, 36
  neurotoxicity 22
  reproductive system effects 22

Molinate:
  abdominal pain 9(540)
  conjunctivitis 9(540)
  diarrhea 9(540)
  fever 9(540)
  nausea 9(540)
  postnatal damage 9(540)
  prenatal damage 9(540)
  weakness 9(540)
Vernolate:
  blood coagulation depression 22
  hemorrhage 22

Toxicology
Monothiocarbamates are metabolized to sulfoxides 9(539). They are not cholinesterase inhibitors.

Active Ingredients
The lists labeled A and B below correspond to the health information designated A and B in the discussion of thiocarbamates.

(A)		(B)	
ferbam	thiram	butylate	molinate
maneb	zineb	cycloate	pebulate
metham	ziram	diallate	triallate
nabam		EPTC	vernolate

Toluene

Inert Ingredient

Synonyms: methyl benzene, phenylmethane

Acute Exposure Effects

anemia

anesthesia

anorexia

ataxia

bone marrow changes

BUN elevated

CNS depression and changes

collapse

coma

confusion

dermatitis

diarrhea

dizziness

drowsiness

eye: irritation, corneal lesions,
  visual disturbances

fatigue

hallucinations

headache

hepatomegaly

hippuric acid levels in urine
  elevated and benzoylglucuronates
  present

lethargy

leukopenia

metabolic acidosis with high anion
  gap

metallic taste

muscular weakness

paresthesias (CNS-related)

proteinuria

respiratory: cough, irritation,
  bronchitis, pulmonary edema,
  depression

thrombocytopenia

toluene in blood

tremors

unconsciousness

vertigo

vomiting

Death due to respiratory failure

Chronic Exposure Effects

anemia

anorexia

BUN elevated

drowsiness

hepatomegaly

hippuric acid levels in
  urine elevated

leukopenia

memory loss

nervousness

pallor

rash

renal damage

thrombocytopenia

toluene in blood

Suspected Effects

adrenal hypertrophy 3(3286)

aplastic anemia 3(3289)

cardiac sensitivity 3(3286)

cerebellar dystropy 3(3286)

β- and γ-globulin and lipoprotein
  levels elevated 3(3286)

hepatic damage 3(3286)

learning capacity decreased 3(3288)

mutagenesis 3(3289), 7(252), 27

neural dystrophy 3(3286)

phagocytic activity of leukocytes
  depressed 3(3286)

plasma hydrocorticoid elevation
  3(3286)

prenatal damage 27

serum albumin depression 3(3286)

Toxicology
Toluene is a fat solvent that causes CNS dysfunction and the destruction of other tissues. It inhibits mitochondrial oxidative phosphorylation. Toulene is oxidized to benzoic acid and conjugated with glycine to form hippuric acid, or with glucuronic acid to yield benzoylglucuronates. Both are excreted in the urine.

Additional Information
Toulene is often contaminated with benzene (see Benzene).

Triazines ——————————————————————————

Class of Active Ingredients

Use: algicides, fungicides, herbicides

Exposure Effects

abdominal pain
adrenal function
  impaired
anemia
dermatitis

diarrhea
eye irritation
mucous membrane
  irritation
nausea

thiamine and
  riboflavin function
  disturbed
vomiting

Suspected Effects

Anilazine:

adrenal degeneration 23
brain degeneration 23
dermal sensitization 23
hepatic degeneration 23
myocardial degeneration 23
renal degeneration 23

Atrazine:

adrenal degeneration 23
anorexia 23
ataxia 1, 23
brain edema and dystrophy 9(563)
cardiac dilation 9(563)
CNS excitation followed by
  depression 9(562)
convulsions 1
erythema 9(562)
eye: conjunctivitis, exophthalmia,
  corneal opacity, iritis 23
growth retardation 9(562), 22
hematocrit depression 22
hemoglobin depression 22
hepatic hemorrhage 9(563)
hypothermia 9(562)
mutagenesis 9(563)
ovarian hemorrhage 23
paralysis 9(563)
prenatal damage 9(563)
renal damage 9(563)
respiratory: hemorrhage, edema,
  pneumonia, bronchitis,
  bradypnea, dyspnea, hyperpnea
  9(562, 563), 23
salivation 23
spasm 9(562)
spleen hemorrhage 9(563)
tremor 23

Suspected Effects (*continued*)

Propazine:
   body weight depression 22
   carcinogenesis 22
   hepatic damage 9(564)
   leukopenia 9(564)

Simazine:
   ataxia 9(564), 23
   carcinogenesis 23
   convulsions 9(564)
   cyanosis 9(564)
   dyspnea 23
   miosis 23
   paralysis 23
   ptosis 23
   tearing 23
   tremor 9(564)
   weakness 9(564)

Toxicology
Triazines may disturb the metabolism of thiamine and riboflavin. They may concentrate and accumulate in the fat of humans and animals.

Active Ingredients

ametryn	hexazinone	propazine
anilazine	isomethiozin	simazine
atraton	methoprotryne	simetryn
atrazine	metribuzin	terbuthylazine
aziprotryne	prometon	terbutryn
cyanazine	prometryn	trietazine
desmetryn		

Triforine ─────────────────────

Active Ingredient

Use: herbicide

Acute Exposure Effects

collapse

depression

dermal irritation

hepatic damage

renal damage

respiratory irritation

weakness

Chronic Exposure Effects

Chronic effects may occur, but no data were found.

Suspected Effects

prenatal damage 23

siderosis 23

Ureas ——————————————————————————

Class of Active Ingredients

Use: defoliants, herbicides, insecticides, rodenticides

Acute Exposure Effects

abdominal distress	diarrhea	nausea
anemia	eye irritation	vomiting
dermal irritation	mucous membrane irritation	

Chronic Exposure Effects

Chronic effects may occur, but no data were found.

Additional Exposure Effects of Pyriminil

anorexia
ataxia
autonomic impairment
bladder dystonia
bowel dystonia
cardiac arrhythmias and ischemia
cerebral edema
chest pain
chills
coma
confusion
dehydration
diabetogenesis
dysphagia
dysphasia
EEG changes
encephalopathy
eye: mydriasis, nystagmus
glycosuria
hypoglycemia followed by
    hyperglycemia and glucose
    intolerance

hypotension (postural)
hypothermia
ketosis
lassitude
motor hyperactivity
muscle weakness
pancreatic damage
paresthesias
peripheral neuropathy
plantar hyperesthesia
polyuria
seizures
tremor

Death due to respiratory failure,
    cardiovascular collapse, or
    ketoacidosis

Suspected Effects

Diflubenzuron:
  carcinogenesis 22
  hemoglobin effects 22
  testosterone depression 22

Diuron:
  carcinogenesis 27
  cyanosis 22
  growth reduction 22, 23
  hemosiderosis 23
  methemoglobinemia 23
  mutagenesis 27
  prenatal damage 27
  red blood cell destruction 22
  splenic damage 23

Fluometuron:
  carcinogenesis 22
  mutagenesis 22

Linuron:
  bone marrow changes 22
  carcinogenesis 22
  exophthalmos 23
  hemorrhagic lungs 23
  mutagenesis 22, 27
  prenatal damage 22, 23
  ptosis 23
  salivation 23
  splenic changes 22
  tearing 22
  weight loss 23

Monuron:
  carcinogenesis 5(392)

Toxicology

Ureas are metabolized via degradation reactions involving N-dealkylation, N-dealkoxylation, ring hydroxylation, oxidation of ring substitutes, and aniline formation by hydrolysis of urea. Polar and acidic metabolites formed by oxidation reactions react further to form diverse conjugates. Substituted ureas can induce or inhibit microsomal enzymes.

Pyriminil poisons β cells of the pancreas causing diabetes mellitus.

Active Ingredients

chlorbromuron	fluometuron	monuron
chloroxuron	isoproturon	neburon
chlortoluron	linuron	pyriminil
difenoxuron	methabenzthiazuron	siduron
diflubenzuron	metobromuron	tebuthiuron
diuron	metoxuron	tetrafluoron
fenuron	monolinuron	thidiazuron

Varnish Makers' and Painters' Naptha ─────────

Inert Ingredient

> **Composition:** xylenes, ethyl benzene, cumene, toluene (usually), benzene (usually), and pyridine (usually)
>   **Synonyms:** V M & P

Acute Exposure Effects

ataxia	mucous membrane	unconsciousness
coma	irritation	vomiting
CNS depression	mydriasis	weakness
conjunctivitis	nausea	
convulsions	olfactory fatigue	Death due to respiratory
dermatitis	respiratory: coughing,	failure
dizziness	irritation, dyspnea	
drowsiness	bronchial	
fatigue	pneumonia,	
headache	depression	
hyperactivity		

Chronic Exposure Effects

anemia	nervousness	proteinuria
dizziness	pain in limbs	weakness
hematuria	paresthesia	weight loss

Suspected Effects

alkaline phosphatase activity increased 3(3377)	neutrophilia 3(3377)
bile duct proliferation 24(87)	preventricular contractions 24(46)
hepatic congestion 24(87)	reticulocytosis 3(3377)
lymphopenia 3(3377)	SGOT depression 3(3377)

Toxicology

Varnish Makers' and Painters' Naphtha is a fat solvent that causes CNS dysfunction and destruction of tissues. The effects attributable to xylene, benzene, toluene, and pyridine can be found under their respective listings in this book.

Xylene ────────────────────────────────────

Active and Inert Ingredient

> **Composition:** The composition of xylene may include a mixture of ortho, para, and meta isomers, ethylbenzene, toluene, trimethylbenzene, phenol, thiophene, pyridine, and nonaromatic hydrocarbons
>
> **Use:** insecticide

Acute Exposure Effects

abdominal pain
amnesia
anemia
anesthesia
anorexia
ataxia
brain hemorrhage
cardiac stress
CNS excitation and depression
coma
confusion
convulsions
dermal: burns, flushing, dermatitis, eczema
dizziness
drowsiness
euphoria
eye: irritation, corneal microvesiculation, disturbed vision, conjunctivitis
headache
hepatic injury
hoarseness
hyperreflexia
hypothermia
irritability
leukocytosis
methylhippuric and toluic acids in urine
mucous membrane irritation and lesions
narcosis
nausea
paresthesia
renal injury
respiratory: dyspnea, coughing, bradypnea, congestion, pneumonitis, edema, hemorrhage, substernal pain
restlessness
salivation
tinnitus
tremor
unconsciousness
vertigo
vomiting
xylene in expired air and blood

Death due to respiratory, hepatic, or renal failure, or ventricular fibrillation

Chronic Exposure Effects

anorexia
apprehension
bone marrow hyperplasia
CNS excitation followed by depression
dermatitis
drowsiness
dyspnea
eye: injury, conjunctivitis
flatulence
GI pain
headache
hepatic: hepatomegaly, necrosis
memory impairment

Chronic Exposure Effects (*continued*)

methylhippuric and toluic acids in urine

mucosal hemorrhage

nausea

nephrosis

nervousness

pallor

paresthesia

red blood cell and white blood cell abnormalities

tremor

vertigo

weakness

thrombocytosis

Suspected Effects

cholinesterase depression 3(3297)

epilepsy (latent) 7(252)

fatty liver 27

hyperplasia (general) 9(123)

mutagenesis 27

prenatal damage 5(168), 27

reproductive system effects 5(343)

Toxicology

Xylene is a fat solvent that causes CNS dysfunction and destruction of other tissues. Oxygenated metabolites produced in the lung may cause pulmonary edema through cellular necrosis. Xylene is metabolized by the cytochrome P-450 system. Red blood cell and white blood cell abnormalities may be due to benzene contamination (see Benzene). Effects may also be due to the presence of other contaminants (see Composition). Also, see Toluene, Phenol, Pyridine and Petroleum Distillates.

Appendix 1

Glossary of Selected Terms

Pesticide Terms

Active ingredient: usually means a single pesticidally active chemical (e.g., parathion). It may also refer to a group of related chemicals that may or may not be isomers (e.g., heptachlor). They are listed on product labels under "active ingredients." Synonym: common name or chemical name.

Chemical name: specific chemical identity of an active or inert ingredient (e.g, *O,O*-diethyl *O-p*-nitrophenyl phosphorothioate is the chemical name of parathion).

Class of active ingredients: ingredients that are grouped together because of their similar chemical structure, toxic mechanism, and health effects (e.g., organophosphates).

Common name: see Active ingredient.

Inert ingredient: solvents, dusts, fillers, or other compounds used in formulating pesticides. Inert ingredients have no pesticidal activity in certain products. Some chemicals are inert in one product and active in others. For example, in a herbicide, an ingredient would be inert if it was not damaging to plants, even though it may be active as an insecticide. Therefore, it is listed as an active ingredient in insecticides but is considered an inert ingredient in herbicides. The names of inert ingredients do not appear on the product label and are considered trade secrets by the manufacturer (e.g., benzene).

Pesticide: specific mixture of active and inert ingredients (e.g., Ortho Home Orchard Spray®).

Pesticide ingredients: active and inert ingredients.

Product name: name given a pesticide product by a manufacturer, distributor, or retailer. It appears on the front of the label (e.g., Ortho Home Orchard Spray®). Synonym: trade name.

Trade name: see product name.

Medical Terms

Mucous membrane effects: effects on the epithelial tissue covering internal organs of the body. The phrase most commonly refers to the mouth, esophagus, trachea, bronchi, and nose which are frequently affected following pesticide exposures, e.g., nasal or bronchial irritation.

Postnatal effects: effects that occur after birth but result from prenatal exposure, e.g., learning disorders, failure to thrive.

Prenatal effects: effects that occur prior to birth and cause the offspring to deviate from the norm. This may include teratogenesis, biochemical alterations, somatic or germ cell modifications, in utero growth retardation, or death. They may not be discernible until after birth.

Reproductive system effects: effects on the reproductive system distinct from the offspring, e.g., testicular atrophy, uterine bleeding.

Appendix 2

Freedom of Information Requests

This book contains some health effects data obtained from the United States Environmental Protection Agency Office of Pesticide Programs, Information Services Branch, Freedom of Information Office. The documents provided were of two types:

Tox One-liners (reference 23). These are brief summaries of the results of animal studies that were submitted by the pesticide manufacturers to U.S.E.P.A. for purposes of registration and tolerance setting.

Surveillance Indices (reference 22). These are summaries of data on pesticide composition, use, food residue tolerances, ecologic effects, and health effects.

These documents do not cover all pesticides, nor do they include all available information on a pesticide. They are useful because they contain health effects data that are not available in the open literature. In the case of newer pesticides, they may be the only source of information.

The results of many health effects studies supplied by pesticide manufacturers to the government were unavailable to the public until 1982. At that time injunctions obtained by the manufacturers, which had prevented the release of study results, were lifted. Results of these studies include information on health effects that was not available in the open literature, and, in the case of new pesticides, was often the only data in existence. While we have obtained some data on over 200 active ingredients, there is a large volume of information that could be useful to health workers that has not yet been released or openly reviewed. The release of most remaining health data was made possible by a June 1984 Supreme Court decision.

For those wishing to request information, the address of the Freedom of Information Office is given below. It is advisable to request a specific type of information on a pesticide, e.g., chronic animal toxicity study results, rather than making a general request, e.g., all the information on acephate. Proprietary information will not be supplied. A major difficulty in obtaining information through the Freedom of Information Act is that requests must be made for specific documents in most cases. It may be difficult to determine if specific information exists and how it is referred to by the government agency. Your government representative or the congressional committee that oversees the agency may be of assistance in this matter.

To obtain information on pesticides, direct inquiries to the following:

U.S.E.P.A.
Office of Pesticide Programs
Information Services Branch
Information Services Section
Freedom of Information Office (A101)
401 M. St., N.W.
Washington, D.C. 20460

Appendix 3

Canceled Pesticides: All Uses (U.S.)

Pesticide	Year Canceled	Effects
arsenic trioxide	1977	M, O, T
BHC	1978	O
bufencarb		
butachlor		
chloranil	1977	O
chlordecone (Kepone®)	1977	O
chloronitropropane		
copper acetoarsenite	1977	M, O, T
copper arsenate (basic)	1977	O
cyprazine		
DDD (TDE)	1971	E
EGT		
erbon	1980	O, R, T
nitralin		
OMPA	1976	O
ovex		
phenarsazine chloride	1977	
pirimicarb		
profluralin		
safrole	1977	M, O
Strobane®	1976	O
TCBC		
Trysben®	1978	O

M = Mutagenesis E = ecologic problems
O = oncogenesis R = reproductive effects
T = teratogenesis

Abstracted from: USEPA, Office of Pesticide Programs, Status Report of RPAR, Special Review, Registration Standards, and Data Call In Programs, September, 1983.

Appendix 4

Canceled Pesticides: Some or Most Uses (U.S.)

Pesticide	Year Canceled	Effects
acrylonitrile	1978	N, O, T
aldrin	1974	E, O
amitraz	1979	O
benzene		B, M, O
chlordane	1974	E, O
DBCP (dibromochloropropane)		M, O, R
DDT	1972	E
dieldrin	1974	E, O
endrin	1979	E, O, T
heptachlor	1974	E, O
isocyanurates		K
lindane	1983	O, R, T
mirex	1976	E
monuron	1977	O
Perthane® (ethylan)	1980	O
pronamide	1979	O
sodium arsenite	1978	M, O, T
strychnine	1983	E
toxaphene	1982	E, O

N = neurotoxicity B = blood disorders
O = oncogenesis   M = mutagenesis
T = teratogenesis   R = reproductive effects
E = ecologic problems K = kidney effects

Abstracted from: USEPA, Office of Pesticide Programs, Status Report on RPAR, Special Review, Registration Standards, and Data Call In Programs, September, 1983.

Appendix 5

Suspended Pesticides (U.S.) Under Consideration for Possible Cancelation

Pesticide	Year Suspended	Effects
ethylene dibromide (EDB)	1983	M, O, T
maleic hydrazide	1981	M, O, R
Silvex® (2,4,5-TP)	1979	O, R, T
2,4,5-T	1979	O, R, T
TEPP		
tetradifon		

M = mutagenesis R = reproductive effects
O = oncogenesis T = teratogenesis

Abstracted from: USEPA, Office of Pesticide Programs, Status Report on RPAR, Special Review, Registration Standards, and Data Call In Programs, September, 1983.

References Cited

1. American Conference of Governmental Industrial Hygienists: Documentation of the Threshold Limit Values, Cincinnati, 1980.
2. Chambers J. E., Yarbrough, J. (eds): Effects of Chronic Exposure to Pesticides on Animal Systems. Raven, New York, 1982.
3. Clayton, G. D., Clayton, F. E. (eds): Patty's Industrial Hygiene and Toxicology, 3rd edition, Volumes 2A, 2B, 2C. Wiley, New York, 1982.
4. Council on Environmental Quality: Chemical Hazards to Human Reproduction. USGPO, Washington, 1981.
5. Doull, J., Klassen, C. D., Amdur, M. O. (eds): Casarett and Doull's Toxicology The Basic Science of Poisons, 2nd edition. Macmillan, New York, 1980.
6. Esposito, M. P., Tierman, T. D., Dryden, F. E.: Dioxins. Cincinnati, EPA, 1980.
7. Finkel, A. J.: Hamilton and Hardy's Industrial Toxicology, 4th edition. Wright, Boston, 1983.
8. Gosselin, R. E., Hodge, H. C., Smith, R. P., Gleason, M. N.: Clinical Toxicology of Commercial Products, 4th edition. Williams & Wilkins, Baltimore, 1976.
9. Hayes, W. H.: Pesticides Studied in Man. Williams & Wilkins, Baltimore, 1982.
10. International Agency for Research on Cancer: IARC Monographs on the Evaluation of Carcinogenic Risk of Chemicals to Man, Carbamates, Thiocarbamates, and Carbazides. Volume 12: WHO, Lyon, 1976.
11. International Agency for Research on Cancer, IARC Monographs on the Evaluation of Carcinogenic Risk of Chemicals to Man, Miscellaneous Pesticides, Volume 30, WHO, Lyon, 1983.
12. International Agency for Research on Cancer: IARC Monographs on the Evaluation of Carcinogenic Risk of Chemicals to Man, Some Halogenated Hydrocarbons, Volume 20: WHO, Lyon, 1979.
13. Kenaja, E. E.: Toxicology and residue data useful in the environmental evaluation of dalapon. Residue Rev 53:109–151, 1974.
14. Key, M. M., Henschel, A. F., Butler, J., Ligo, R. N., Tabershaw, I. R., Ede, L. (eds): Occupational Diseases A Guide to Their Recognition. USGPO, Washington, 1977.
15. Morgan, D. P.: Recognition and Management of Pesticide Poisoning, 3rd edition, USGPO, Washington, 1982.
16. Neal, R. A. Microsomal metabolism of thiono-sulfur compounds: mechanisms and toxicological significance. Rev Biochem Toxicol 2:131–171, 1980.
17. Patty, F. A. (ed): Industrial Hygiene and Toxicology, 2nd edition. Interscience, New York, 1958.
18. Sax NI: Dangerous Properties of Industrial Materials, 5th edition. Van Nostrand Reinhold, New York, 1979.
19. Shiau, S. Y., Huff, R. A., Wells, B. C., Felkner, I. C.: Mutagenicity and DNA-damaging activity for several pesticides tested with *Bacillus subtilis* mutants. Mutat Res 71:169–179, 1980.

20. Sittig M: Handbook of Toxic and Hazardous Chemicals. Noyes, Park Ridge, New Jersey, 1981.
21. Sittig, M. (ed): Pesticide Manufacturing and Toxic Materials Control Encyclopedia. Noyes, Park Ridge, New Jersey, 1980.
22. Surveillance indices: See Appendix 2.
23. Tox one-liners: See Appendix 2.
24. USDHEW, PHS, CDC, NIOSH: Criteria for a recommended standard: Occupational Exposure to Refined Petroleum Solvents. USGPO, Washington, 1977.
25. USDHHS/USDOL, NIOSH, OSHA: Occupational Health Guidelines for Chemical Hazards, NIOSH, 1981.
26. USDHHS, PHS, CDC, NIOSH: Registry of Toxic Effects of Chemical Substances. USGPO, Washington, 1980.
27. USDHHS, PHS, CDC, NIOSH: Registry of Toxic Effects of Chemical Substances. USGPO, Washington, 1983.
28. USDHHS: Third Annual Report on Carcinogenesis. USGPO, Washington, 1982.
29. USEPA: Pesticide Registration Standard for Carboxin, NTIS PB82-131731, 1981.
30. USEPA: Pesticide Registration Standard for Chloramben, NTIS PB82-134347, 1981.
31. USEPA: Pesticide Registration Standard for Isopropalin, NTIS PB82-131293, 1981.
32. USEPA: Pesticide Registration Standard for Metalaxyl, NTIS PB82-172297, 1981.
33. USEPA: Pesticide Registration Standard for Methomyl, NTIS PB82-180738, 1981.
34. USEPA: Pesticide Registration Standard for Naphthaleneacetic Acid, NTIS PB82-131145, 1981.
35. USEPA: Pesticide Registration Standard for OBPA, NTIS PB82-172271, 1981.
36. Vettorazzi, G.: International Regulatory Aspects for Pesticide Chemicals, Volume 1, Toxicity Profiles. CRC, Boca Raton, Florida, 1979.
37. Wiltrout, R. W., Ercegovich, C. D., Ceglowski, W. S.: Humoral immunity in mice following oral administration of selected pesticides. Bull. Environ. Contam Toxicol 20:423–431, 1978.

References Consulted and Suggested

American Conference of Governmental Industrial Hygienists: Documentation of the Threshold Limit Values, Cincinnati, 1980.

Berg, G. L. (ed), Farm Chemicals Handbook, Meister Pub. Co, Willoughby, Ohio, 1983.

Caswell, R. L., Debold, K. J., Gilbert, L. S. (eds): Pesticide Handbook (Entoma), 29th edition. Entomological Society of America, College Park, Maryland, 1981.

Clayton, G. D., Clayton, F. E. (eds): Patty's Industrial Hygiene and Toxicology, 3rd edition, Volumes 2A, 2B, 2C. Wiley, New York, 1982.

Council on Environmental Quality: Chemical Hazards to Human Reproduction. USGPO, Washington, 1981.

Doull, J., Klassen, C. D., Amdur, M. O. (eds): Casarett and Doull's Toxicology The Basic Science of Poisons, 2nd edition. Macmillan, New York, 1980.

Driesbach, R. H.: Handbook of Poisoning: Diagnosis and Treatment, 7th edition. Lange, Los Altos, California, 1971.

Finkel, A. J.: Hamilton and Hardy's Industrial Toxicology, 4th edition. Wright, Boston, 1983.

Gosselin, R. E., Hodge, H. C., Smith, R. P., Gleason, M. N.: Clinical Toxicology of Commercial Products, 4th edition. Williams & Wilkins, Baltimore, 1976.

Hayes, W. H.: Pesticides Studied in Man. William & Wilkins, Baltimore, 1982.

Key, M. M., Henschel, A. F., Butler, J., Ligo, R. N., Tabershaw, I. R., Ede, L. (eds): Occupational Diseases: A Guide to Their Recognition. USGPO, Washington, 1977.

Lefevre, M. J.: First Aid Manual for Chemical Accidents. Dowden Hutchinson and Ross, Stroudsburg, Pennsylvania, 1980.

Morgan, D. P.: Recognition and Management of Pesticide Poisoning, 3rd edition. USGPO, Washington, 1982.

Sax, N. I.: Cancer Causing Chemicals. Van Nostrand Reinhold, New York, 1981.

Sax, N. I.: Dangerous Properties of Industrial Materials, 5th edition. Van Nostrand Reinhold, New York, 1979.

Sittig, M.: Handbook of Toxic and Hazardous Chemicals. Noyes, Park Ridge, New Jersey, 1981.

Sittig, M. (ed): Pesticide Manufacturing and Toxic Materials Control Encyclopedia. Noyes, Park Ridge, New Jersey, 1980.

USDHHS/USDOL, NIOSH, OSHA: Occupational Health Guidelines for Chemical Hazards, NIOSH, 1981.

USDHHS, PHS, CDC, NIOSH: Registry of Toxic Effects of Chemical Substances. USGPO, Washington, 1983.

USDHHS: Third Annual Report on Carcinogenesis. USGPO, Washington, 1982.

Weiss, G. (ed): Hazardous Chemicals Data Book. Noyes, Park Ridge, New Jersey, 1980.

Windholz, M., Budavari, S., Stroumtsos, L. Y., Fertig, M. N. (eds) The Merck Index. Merck, Rahway, New Jersey, 1976.

Series

International Agency for Research on Cancer, IARC Monographs on the Evaluation of the Carcinogenic Risk of Chemicals to Humans, IARC, Lyon.
USDHHS, PHS, CDC, NIOSH: Criteria for Recommended Standards, USGPO, Washington, D.C.
USEPA: Pesticide Registration Standards, NTIS or USGPO, Washington, D.C.
USEPA: Surveillance Indices, Freedom of Information Office, USEPA Office of Pesticide Programs. See Appendix 2.
USEPA: Tox One-liners, Freedom of Information Office, USEPA Office of Pesticide Programs. See Appendix 2.
WHO: Pesticide Residue Series, WHO, Geneva

Journals

Annals of Occupational Hygiene
Archives of Environmental Contamination and Toxicology
Archives of Environmental Health
British Journal of Industrial Medicine
Bulletin of Environmental Contamination Toxicology
Bulletin of the National Clearinghouse of Poison Control Centers
Food and Cosmetic Toxicology
Journal of Industrial Hygiene Toxicology
Residue Reviews
Toxicology and Applied Pharmacology
Specific pesticides can be researched through the use of Pesticide Abstracts, a citation index.

Data Bases

TOXLINE/TOXBACK	CANCER LIT	POISINDEX
CSIN	CTCP	RTECS
MEDLINE	EMIC	TDB
PESTAB	ETIC	

Index

This index contains an alphabetical list of all pesticide ingredients and classes of ingredients discussed in this book. Active and inert ingredient names have been used rather than chemical names because ingredients are usually referred to, both on the labels and in discussions of health effects, by their active or inert ingredient names. Often the chemical name is the same as the active ingredient name, e.g., carbon tetrachloride.

Trade names have been included only if they are commonly used in place of the active ingredient name. Trade names are capitalized and the symbol ® follows the names.

Frequently used synonyms are included in this index. The synonyms are followed, in parentheses, by the active ingredient name which will usually appear on a label, or in the case of an inert ingredient, by the most commonly used inert ingredient name. For example, chlorophenothane is a synonym for the more commonly used active ingredient name DDT. It appears as follows in the index: chlorophenothane (DDT).

The number following each entry refers to the page where the health discussion for that ingredient begins. The index is set up strictly alphabetically, regardless of how names are divided.

For example: ethyl acetate
               ethylene glycol
               ethylmercuric salicylate
               ethyl parathion

The designations of chemical position preceding a name are not used as the first letter of the name in the alphabetization of the index. For example, *O*-dichlorobenzene is listed under "d" for dichlorobenzene.